Cristy Lane

Her life had been a roller coaster of joy and sorrow, and many times she had wondered how she would make it through the next day. There were times when she had needed a strength from beyond herself . . . *Please, sweet Jesus, help me* . . . And He had, for her faith had been deeply rooted in her since her childhood. That had been a long time ago. She had called on God many times since then. Yet that was all inward, private between her and God. She would like to express to others—but she didn't know how—the way she really felt. Now she had finally found one song that could do it for her. The lyrics summed up her life—and how, over the years, she had learned to live it . . .

One Day at a Time

"With all the music that has come and gone, 'One Day at a Time' is still my number one request."
—"Jaybird" Drennan, WSLR-Radio, Akron, Ohio

"Cristy Lane's biography brings a lump to your throat." —*The Tribune-Democrat*

Cristy Lane
One Day at a Time

Lee Stoller
with Pete Chaney

St. Martin's Press • *LS*
New York

*This book is true, but certain names have been changed and some conver-
sations paraphrased in order to avoid intrusion on the privacy of certain
individuals.*

CRISTY LANE: ONE DAY AT A TIME

Copyright © 1983 by Lee Stoller

Printed in the United States of America

First St. Martin's Press mass market edition/September 1986

ISBN: 0-312-90415-0
Can. ISBN: 0-312-90416-9

10 9 8 7 6 5 4 3 2 1

To my Wife: Cristy

I HAD A DREAM, AND I DO BELIEVE IN ANGELS.
I THANK GOD AND YOU FOR MY LIFE.
FOR BEING THERE WHEN I NEEDED YOU MOST.
FOR GIVING ME THE STRENGTH TO FACE EACH DAY.
AND FOR MAKING MY DREAM COME TRUE, "ONE DAY AT A TIME."

LOVE FOREVER,
Lee

1

She lived in the world of nine-year-olds,
cushioned by day dreams, make-believe,
rag dolls. Christmas was coming. And so
was her first great heartbreak.

She was Ellie Johnston then, not the Cristy Lane
of today. She didn't know she wasn't well off. She
lived in East Peoria, Illinois. And she had a dream.
A typical nine-year-old girl's dream . . . of a brand-
new doll all her very own.

The one in the store window downtown.

Ellie Johnston had never had a brand-new doll
before. Most of her toys—and all her dolls—were
well-used by older sisters long before her fingers
touched them. But this Christmas it *could* be different. She *might* possess the doll of her dreams.

The brand-new doll. The one no one else had
loved before her . . . For days now it had beckoned
to her from the store window. It was dressed in
beautiful, shining silk. It sat beside a sign that said:
"Shake me, I rattle. Squeeze me, I cry." It was irre-
sistible.

In the days before Christmas, Ellie made several

trips to the store to look with yearning. The price was $2.00—beyond the reach of her meager savings. But each trip she carried all the money she had anyway—pennies, nickels, and dimes wrapped carefully in a handkerchief. Maybe a miracle.

The miracle happened two days before Christmas. The big placard in the store window announced that all toys were on sale. Ellie wiped the snow from the corner of the window to see the price of the doll. Her doll.

$1.25.

Her savings were enough.

She thought.

The clerk brought the doll from the window and placed it on the counter, inches from Ellie's excited eyes. Ellie handed her the handkerchief, and the clerk began to count the change.

$1.20. $1.21. $1.22. $1.23. $1.24. The handkerchief was empty.

"You're a penny shy," the impassive clerk said.

"Can I go home and get the other penny? Will you hold it for me?"

"We hold no merchandise. If it's here when you get back, fine. Otherwise, someone else will buy it. Our toys are moving fast on sale."

The clerk's voice was cold . . . cold as the snow falling outside, Ellie thought. The doll still smiled at her, but now it seemed far away. It would go to someone else. Someone better. She, Ellie, was not worthy. Not part of the big world. Not good enough.

Slowly she picked up the change from the counter. The clerk's eyes were on her, but there was no feeling in them. The clerk didn't care. She, Ellie, was nothing.

She turned away from the counter dejected. For reasons that were not clear to her she walked slowly over to the household wares counter nearby and picked out a salt and pepper shaker set for her mother for Christmas. It took all of her money except for a quarter and some pennies. She spent the pennies on lollipops. Somehow they didn't taste as good as she thought they would.

She still had a quarter left.

The snow was falling heavier when she started home. She made her way through the scurrying adult shoppers tramping the icy white sidewalk. Ahead of her, seated on the curb, was a beggar bundled against the cold, his tin cup in a shivering hand.

People passed him by, busy with their own lives. Ellie, feeling his misery, tried to look away. Nobody wanted him, either. He, too, was unworthy. Not part of the big world. Not good enough. A nothing . . .

Her eyes came back to him, nearer now. Resolutely she walked past, then hesitated . . . and looked back.

He seemed so all alone.

Quickly Ellie turned back to him, unravelled that last quarter from her handkerchief, and dropped it with a clatter into the empty cup.

She did not feel better. She had not done it for that reason. She hurried toward home. She wanted to cry her heart out, but she didn't. In the crowded street she was alone.

She hurried, hearing as nine-year-olds will, the silent music of the snow.

That was the first heartbreak of the girl who would one day be Cristy Lane. It would not be the last. Before the fairy godmother, Fame, touched her with the golden wand she would know at first hand the sorrows about which country music—the most typical of American art forms—sings. And to endure her sorrows she would need the strength of that other typical American music, gospel.

Typical. She was the typical one.

Even from the day of her birth . . .

January 8, 1940. Franklin Delano Roosevelt was in the White House. The Depression was over. Business was booming. Times were good—especially in Peoria, Illinois, the "Ideal American Community." Here was born Eleanor Johnston, the eighth of the twelve children of Andrew and Pansy Johnston.

Well, not exactly in Peoria. Across the river in East Peoria. In the working class section. In the depressed area. Where people were poor. But happy.

Home for the Johnston family was a small white frame house sitting bleakly at 616 South Main Street. It had two bedrooms, a small kitchen, and a living room/dining room combination. There was no inside toilet. You went outside, to a small outhouse in the rear, hard by the tracks of the Peoria and Pekin Union Railroad switchyards.

It was a happy home, though, and even the six other children (one other child had died in infancy) eagerly welcomed the new arrival. Tiny Eleanor, lovingly nicknamed "Ellie" by her father, crawled in secure comfort across the well-worn, spotlessly-scrubbed linoleum floor of the kitchen. Pansy would bend down and pick her up, caressing her softly and whispering soothingly. Andrew would follow, nuzzling the unshaven bristles of his face against the fragile little cheek. The other children would gather round, proclaiming each in turn would be the next to hold her. Whatever was missing in money or luxury in this family was made up for in warmth, love, and closeness. Sharing was something they all took for granted.

Baby Ellie's eager young nose could always smell something good cooking in her mama's kitchen. In addition to being a loving mother and good wife, Pansy was also a skilled and efficient cook. She would take the sparse income Andrew brought home and with it spread a wholesome and tasty dining table. A favorite saying of Andrew was that "Pansy could boil water and make even it taste good."

In the kitchen, before and after meals, was where the children learned of the outside world. Andrew, though a common laborer and thus considered the "black sheep" of his own family, was an avid reader and digested every word of the cherished evening paper. The children would listen as Andrew talked of news events he had heard discussed that day at work. And he would read from the newspaper to anyone who cared to listen.

But also in the kitchen was the small black radio atop the icebox—placed there out of reach of restless and curious young hands. The radio brought the world and outside activity to the Johnston family. And it entertained. Pansy listened to her soap operas while Andrew was at work. "Helen Trent" . . . "Portia Faces Life" . . . "Ma Perkins."

The radio also brought something else:

Music . . .

To the wide-eyed young Ellie the little black box was a fascinating marvel. At first the tiny radio seemed a mile away, a source of multiple voices, strange sounds, and tingling music. As she grew older she enjoyed with the others of her family "Superman" and "Inner Sanctum"—but her real favorite was "The Lucky Strike Hit Parade." The songs stimulated her whole being. Even before her school years she would stand below the radio, the music showering down upon her, and her senses would be tantalized by the sounds coming from the magic box above. Her tiny body would weave and dance to the music. She would hum along with each song. Gradually she learned the words. Then she would harmonize with the singers, quickly memorizing the melody . . . before she was old enough to know what the words meant.

So music became a part of her . . .

Meanwhile, of course, other children were being born into the Johnston family, adding to the feeling of closeness and security for Ellie as each child in his turn was the loved and cuddled baby, then later helped with the new arrivals.

For tiny Ellie Saturday nights were the most fun because of "bath night." Pansy pulled a galvanized tub into the kitchen so that each child could take his turn. There being no hot water heater, Pansy would heat kettles and large pans of water on the wood stove and transfer the steaming contents to the tub, her apron on the handles to protect her hands from the heat. There would be a lot of laughing, giggling, and cavorting. And—to Pansy's dismay—a lot of spilled water.

So Ellie had a warm and secure childhood.

Until Christmas when she was nine.

And until a Sunday when she was ten.

Oddly, it had to do with religion.

Pansy Johnston was a woman of strong moral

values and sent her children often to the Methodist church, accompanying them when her household chores would allow it. Ellie loved church and found the same sense of security there that she did at home.

But this particular Sunday . . .

Ellie was ten years old now. Always a small child, she had grown even prettier. She was, as the saying goes, "a petite beauty," and she had caught the fancy of a neighbor lady, a member of a different denomination than the Johnstons. This particular morning the neighbor dropped by and asked Pansy if she could take Ellie to her church.

Pansy hesitated. Then, thinking it might be good for Ellie to experience new surroundings, she reluctantly agreed.

Still, there was a shadow on her face as she watched Ellie leave, hand in hand with the neighbor lady . . .

Some time later, at the strange church, that small hand was gripping the neighbor lady's even tighter. As a matter of fact, Ellie was holding on with all her might—as if her life depended upon it.

She and the neighbor lady were standing before the preacher of that church, and Ellie was wishing desperately that Pansy had kept her at home.

The preacher was yelling at her.

Only it wasn't like he was a preacher anymore . . . He was a big, terrible monster in a black suit, the very figure of doom. The yelling scared her so much she didn't get the first thing he said to her. Then she did:

"Ellie Johnston! You must repent! You're an evil girl! A sinner! Like everyone else here today! But they have confessed their sins! And they shall see . . . the Kingdom of God!"

Scared as she was, she couldn't help but hear a rhythm in his rising and falling voice . . . the music of doom . . .

He went on, only his voice got louder and louder, and Ellie heard the words less and less. It was like what he was yelling was something that was hot that got hotter. Was this what Hell was like? Ellie could feel the beads of perspiration forming on her forehead, could even, she thought, feel the small wisps of her brown hair turning limp around her braids. Was she melting? In the fires of Hell?

Wildly, she looked around for escape.

Only to have her blue eyes widen with a greater fear.

The people.

They had gone mad.

Not ten feet from Ellie an old, old woman was rolling around on the church floor. Shouting.

A young boy, not much older than herself, was writhing soundlessly in the aisle.

Then . . .

One by one and two by two other members of the congregation joined the old woman and the young boy on the church floor. Moaning. Yelling. Shouting things in an unknown language. Contorted. Frantic.

The world had come to an end.

Nothing like this had ever happened in her Methodist church.

"Ellie Johnston!"

She jumped.

Her head snapped back sharply as she turned to face the angry man with the booming voice.

"How dare you defy the Lord your God! Unless you repent this day you shall not enter the Kingdom of Heaven! You will be damned for all eternity! Cast into the fiery pit of Hell! A worthless sinner! Repent!"

Ellie was too scared to even speak, much less repent. That is, if she had known what "repent" meant. Why was this man yelling at her? What had she done that was so awful? How had she sinned? She wanted to run and hide. Nothing like this had ever happened in the Methodist church. There she had always felt as warm and secure as in her own home . . . felt as though God and Jesus loved her and wanted her to be happy. Here before this powerful figure who seemed to have some kind of special telephone line to God and sin—particularly sin— she felt small and unworthy.

More unworthy now than when she had failed to get the doll in the store window.

Only this time there was not even the silent

music of the falling snow . . . Only a rising storm of confused and distorted sound . . .

In that storm she felt something within her quietly die.

(Years later the adult Cristy Lane would understand that different persons have different ways to approach their Maker, and that the great words of religion like "repentance" and "conviction" and "sin" may sometimes be presented by one person in ways that seem strange to another. But that would be years later. This Sunday Ellie Johnston, who up to this time had known the church only as a place of love and security, was not prepared for what she experienced.)

The second of the three childhood events that would alter Ellie's life had just occurred.

The third was four years away.

Meanwhile . . .

2

C at got your tongue?"

Ellie glanced up into her father's smiling eyes. It was that same Sunday evening. Ever since she had come home from the neighbor lady's church Ellie had been quiet. Too quiet. Even at the supper table, with its bountiful Sunday regular of roast and potatoes, she had been quiet. More than that. She had merely stared at her plate, not eating. This had concerned her mother Pansy greatly. Ellie was tiny for a 10-year-old, weighing barely 40 pounds. Pansy certainly didn't want her to lose any of what little weight she did possess. She asked Ellie what was wrong. It was normal for this close-knit family to share its troubles around the table, so they all listened as Ellie tried to explain what had happened at the services that day. But in her excitement of relating the events her habit of rapid speech delivery combined with her pronounced lisp to make it next to impossible to express what she wanted to tell them. If only she could explain to all of them how she felt inside! She gave up trying and sat staring at her food, choking back tears, feeling empty and alone. Pansy watched her, thinking of the handicap of the lisp and silently worrying about being able to get Ellie into special speech classes before permanent damage was done. But Andrew . . .

Andrew had the feeling, rightly or wrongly, that he knew what was going on in his little girl's mind. He had looked over at her tiny, forlorn face. He loved that little girl. Not unlike himself, she was a dreamer.

A dreamer . . .

To almost all of the world around him Andrew was simply a common laborer at the Herschel Manufacturing Company, one of the faceless many on the farm machinery assembly lines. Not even a particularly successful worker. The expanded work at the plant, brought on by the war in Europe and the end of the Depression, had increased his weekly pay envelope, and he could now feed and clothe his family a little better. But there was nothing left for luxuries. Not even a car. He did not own one. He would never own one. And to the day he died he would walk to work—and walk back.

A dreamer?

Well, there was the beer. It was not that it was a great big problem. Not big enough for Pansy to complain, though many were the nights when Andrew would walk in the door carrying his bamboo fishing pole, a string of fish he had caught on the banks of the Illinois River—and that mischievous, ever-present grin on his face. He always carried beer with him when he went fishing, and the more he drank the wider the grin became. Pansy had never made much fuss over his drinking. It never seemed to affect his work, and he was never violent toward her or the children. But there had been many nights when she had guided him gently to their room and into bed. And both of them knew there would be many more in the future.

But drinking beer does not make a man a dreamer.

There was the other thing.

Andrew's artistic talent.

He had once contemplated becoming an artist. He had the ability. He had received many compliments on his sketches, sketches he had never been able to keep himself from drawing. He had even had the dream . . . a career in oils . . . or watercolors . . . or acrylics . . . A sweet and distant dream.

But . . .

He had married Pansy, and one child after another had come along, and their needs had kept him rooted to his labor. A steady income was needed to feed these growing bodies, one that a struggling artist could never provide. He hadn't done so bad, though. They had a roof over their heads, food in their mouths, and they all seemed content. All except Ellie, that was. Something beside a simple church service was bothering his little girl tonight. Usually Pansy had to scold her for singing at the table during meals. How she did love to sing! And she was good at it, too. Andrew felt a smile on his lips as he thought of her—ever since he could remember—being fascinated by the small radio on the icebox. He could still see her dancing and singing along with the music, knowing all the words by heart. It seemed to him she must have taken a special pleasure in singing his favorites, the Doris Day and Patti Page hits. Yes, she was always singing— at least until someone in the family told her to shut up. He never shushed her, though. Maybe it was because her singing was like his art . . . part of a dream. Weren't they two of a kind? One day he had even sneaked her out of the house and down to his favorite tavern where he had stood her on the bar and had her sing "Paper Doll" for his cronies. She had looked so cute standing up there on the bar, singing, smiling at everyone. He wished that she was smiling now as she had then . . .

"What's the matter with my little singer tonight?" he said gently. "Cat got your tongue?"

She looked up at him, but her lips did not move. There was pain in her eyes. He wondered what she was thinking . . .

Ellie was thinking how much she wanted to tell this understanding father how lonely and unimportant she felt . . . as if she were nothing at all but a tiny, meaningless speck . . . and how much she hated the feeling. But the words would not come. And she hated that even more. And then she felt even worse when she saw what seemed like a cloud pass across his eyes.

She wanted to cry her heart out.

But she didn't.

At least not in front of the family.

That night she lay in bed trying to read, the one thing she loved to do. Books brought her friends in far-off places, friends that couldn't get close enough to hurt her since they were tucked into the pages of a book.

But try as she would Ellie could not erase the images from her mind: . . . frantic bodies writhing around on the floor of the church . . . the ominous-looking preacher yelling to everyone what a horrible little person she was . . .

She swallowed the lump that was forming in her throat. She didn't want her brothers and sisters to hear her cry. But not only could she not drive the day's thoughts from her mind, she had others . . . from school . . . Her classmates teased her often enough about being small. Too small. Every Monday morning everyone in class was weighed on scales as part of the physical health program. And when Ellie started for the scales . . .

It seemed to her she could still hear the remembered giggling . . . The needle on the face of the dial would barely move when she stepped up. The laughter and taunting of her classmates was as predictable as her small weight and lack of gaining more. If only she were bigger, like the rest! Or if she had pretty clothes! Or if her nose didn't turn up at the tip like it did! Then maybe they wouldn't tease her so much. And maybe the preacher wouldn't have yelled at her the way he had at church today.

But they were only "ifs" . . . and he had yelled.

Suddenly she could hold her tears no longer. She buried her head in the pillow. Outside, close by, a freight train rumbled by, going away . . . going . . .

It was a long time before sleep came to her.

Ellie withdrew deeper within herself. Her lisp, her small frame and stature, her only self-conceived "faults" were all embarrassing to her.

The lisp really wasn't the big thing, but it became the symbol . . . proof that she was unworthy . . . It had made her "cute" when she first began to speak. Now it made her an object of ridicule. She tried to avoid the words that contained an "S" when she spoke because if she used them it sounded like she was whistling. But . . . by the time she was in the sixth grade the lisp had created for her what she considered catastrophic problems. So she spoke out in class only when it was absolutely necessary.

And that didn't help her scholastic standing one bit.

But Pansy, out of love and necessity, finally found a way to finance speech therapy for Ellie. It worked. When she completed this special training, which stressed phonics and syllable pronounciation, Ellie finally mastered the art of perfect diction. Even though she kept her habit of rapid-fire delivery of speech, she was still able to speak with precision and clear enunciation. This was a trait that would stay with her for life.

But she was still reluctant to stray from the immediate environment of her family's circle. It provided security. It posed no threat to her—as did the outside world. She found a haven in reading to fill the void created by her compulsion to stay at home. Like all youngsters she had traded comic books with friends. Now the comic books were replaced with hardcover volumes of romance, intrigue, or ancient history. History was her favorite, but her tastes ran from mysteries to biographies of the great. Her dream world, though—when she could afford it—was at the movies. Here she usually went with her closest and dearest friend, Carol Hatcher. Carol, like Ellie, came from a poor family, and they found that they had a lot in common so their relationship grew. Crying, laughing, loving, they placed themselves in the roles of their screen stars, aching when they ached, smiling when they smiled, crying when they cried. The two girls would stay through several showings of the same film—especially if it starred one of their favorites. Burt Lancaster and Susan Hayward were two such. Two films that particularly touched Ellie and Carol were "I Want to Live" and "I'll Cry Tomorrow." Together, they lived and cried through both.

Together they also went to church. At the services Ellie was often asked by those aware of her talent to sing a solo—or a "special" as some called it—for the congregational services. But here there was a problem. Ellie was acutely aware of her worn and plain hand-me-down dresses. And she was also much too shy to sing in front of an audience. There was an ingenious solution: Ellie sang from behind the curtains. Safe from the eyes of the crowd she felt free in the music and out of harm's way from the crowd. Her voice would ring out, and it would be a moment of glory. After services she would timidly try to avoid the compliments of the congregation, wishing at the moment that both she and her darned and faded old dress were invisible from human eyes. Yet each time she gained a little more confidence.

Until . . .

But that was to come later . . .

Inevitably, of course, she began to mature. But just as she had earlier been embarrassed by her small size, now she was embarrassed by her small breasts. Her first training bra was more a token than a necessity. And since she was already acutely self-conscious about her clothes, she was not prepared for dating.

And, again, there was an incident.

Putting her books into the locker at school one afternoon, she heard two boys on the other side of the locker start talking about her.

"Why don't you ask her for a date?" one said. "She's pretty."

"Naw. Ellie's just a kid. I want a grown-up date."

A "grown-up date"? She wondered what it was. And asked a girl friend. Told what boys expected from a girl on a date, Ellie blushed and determined she didn't want that.

Still, the school years were relatively happy.
Until the night of the teen choir at school.
And even that started off on a high note.
This night was special.
Special!

Ellie was now a sophomore in high school. She was 14 years old, and she had traded in her braids for soft curls. Tonight she was scheduled to sing with the school choir for her first *live* audience— that is, face-to-face and not from behind a curtain.

Before she left home she stopped for one last look at herself in the mirror, and smiled happily at what she saw. She was wearing the most beautiful dress she had ever worn. Pansy had made it over from one of her older sister's dresses, but it looked brand-new. True, the teacher had told them all to wear white dresses, but there hadn't been a white one for Ellie, and this would have to do. After all, the polka dots were small. Hardly noticeable . . .

She made one last effort at patting in place a particularly unruly curl and skipped out of the house, her china-blue eyes sparkling with excitement and anticipation. She had practiced long and hard for this performance. She knew all the songs perfectly.

But, more than that, tonight was *special* . . . in a way she could not explain.

The seats in the school auditorium were already starting to fill when she arrived. She hurried to take her place in line with the rest of her classmates. They all stood quietly behind the red, heavily-worn drapes that separated them from the audience, each waiting his or her turn to be inspected by the teacher. The overhead lights reflected off shoes shined to a high gloss. The rustling of heavily starched skirts filled the air.

Here came the teacher.

Pinched, aquiline nose quivering.

Like a hawk ready to strike. Searching for the tiniest thing wrong . . .

Ellie squeezed her own tiny hands until they hurt, hardly able to contain herself as her turn came and she stepped out into the light for inspection.

Then . . .

The teacher eyed Ellie intently, began to shake her head, and the look on her thin, mean face became one of disgust and contempt. She began sarcastically, her voice low, then gradually rising:

"You don't really think you are going on stage dressed like that, do you?"

"Ma'am?"

"You were told to wear a white dress."

Ellie's timid smile faded, and she bit her lip to fight back the tears welling up in her eyes. She could hear the snickers of her classmates who had always whispered about the clothes she wore.

"It's my sister's dress, ma'am," she stammered, her voice surprisingly clear and melodious despite choking emotion. "We couldn't afford a new one. It's the best my mother had."

"I distinctly said 'an all-white dress'!" the teacher barked.

The snickers of the classmates had stopped. So had the rustling skirts. There was a cold silence on the stage that made Ellie feel more alone than she ever felt in her life.

The teacher's next words seemed even colder: "This won't do at all. You are excused. Someone else will sing your part."

The tears wouldn't stay back now. They blinded Ellie as she turned and stumbled from the stage, through the exit, into the night.

A slow, mocking rain had begun to fall, and in her wild, sobbing flight back home she was soon soaked to the skin, the dress she had thought the most beautiful she had ever worn clinging wetly to her body like the cold fetters of a prisoner.

It was like it had been when she had lost the chance at the doll . . . only now there was no silent music as from the snow, only the words rising and falling in her mind: *I will never go on a stage! They can have their old music! I will never sing again!*

Pansy slipped her own oversized robe over her small daughter's shoulders, dried Ellie's hair, and tried to pat away the tears. "Don't cry anymore, Eleanor," she said comfortingly.

"Why, Mom?" Ellie sobbed. "Why are people the way they are?"

"Some people just don't understand the problems other people have. Or the things they can't help that make them different."

"All I wanted to do was sing with them! They didn't want me . . ."

"Without realizing it, people are sometimes just cruel to one another."

Ellie's brothers and sisters sat quietly around the table, mutely sharing her grief. Andrew, a beer in his hand, sat near the stove, his feet propped up on a pile of wood. His eyes were staring straight ahead, his own pain silent but deep.

Ellie still sobbed. "She wouldn't let me sing! All because of the polka dots on the dress. I thought they wouldn't notice. I just don't want to be part of them anymore."

Pansy put her arms around the frail body and pulled Ellie close. "No, honey, that's not right. Don't let some teacher turn you against something you love to do."

"I don't want to sing in their school choir again. The church choir, either. I don't want to ever sing again."

"No, Ellie. God blessed you with a beautiful voice. Don't turn away from it."

Andrew stirred. "Yes, Ellie. You've got to sing. You have the gift of song. One day, when you sing, people won't care what kind of clothes you're wearing. They'll just want to hear you sing. Don't give up the dream."

Ellie looked from one parent to the other. She said nothing aloud, but in her mind the silent words shouted:

I'll never sing again! Never!

3

L ee Stoller eyed his blind date approvingly. *She was cute.* He would give her that. Soft brown hair. Trusting blue eyes. And, he thought, *A very special way of smiling . . .* Tiny, too. She couldn't be over five feet—if she was that. Probably didn't weigh over a hundred pounds. She was wearing a black sweater and plaid slacks. *Not bad at all,* he finalized, confirming his first impression.

It was one of the few blind dates he had ever accepted. He really didn't need to accept any. No, not Lee Stoller. When he had pulled into the parking lot of the skating rink where they were to meet he had almost decided to pull right back out and forget the whole thing. But now he was glad he hadn't . . .

The friend who had lined up the date made the introductions:

"Lee, this is Ellie Johnston. Ellie, meet Lee Stoller."

She smiled, and again Lee was glad he had kept the date. Despite his experience with women and his very active social life, at the moment he almost stammered in his eagerness to tell her how pleased he was to meet her.

Lee, recently discharged from a two-year hitch in the Marine Corps, possessed the bearing and the self-assurance that generally come with the title "Ex-Marine." He had an ego, too—as Ellie would soon discover. He had gone to work for the P & PU Railroad after his discharge, and nearly all his weekly pay went into a '55 Chevy—and a very "in" wardrobe. Tonight his slacks and sport shirt were new and expensive. He was absolutely certain that the petite young thing standing before him would have to be very impressed.

As they began to glide around the rink, Lee punctuated his conversation with tricky maneuvers on his skates, obviously showing off. His 20-year-old frame, honed by Marine Corps training and exercise, was at a peak of strength and agility. He skated backwards. He made spins. He leaped effortlessly into the air and landed on bent knee. It was a good show, not only for Ellie but also for the other girls at the rink he knew would be looking.

Lee was quite a ladies' man and knew many of the young girls here tonight. They returned his smile and answered his "Hello!" as he skated by. Lee flirted openly with all of them while circling the rink with Ellie, and as a result Ellie's side of their conversation waned.

She was not amused.

Ellie had let Suzie talk her into this blind date. Now she regretted it, wishing right now that she was at home with a good book—where she usually was in the evening. Yes, right from the moment of their introduction to each other she had been somehow turned off by him, and now she was beginning to understand why. Oh, he was handsome, all right. Suzie had told the truth there. He had a round, happy face, and it was continually bursting into an infectious smile. And he had nice clothes . . . which draped a handsome and muscular body . . .

But . . .

Ellie had never met anyone who was so brash. So self-confident.

It was the self-confidence that rankled. It touched a raw nerve in her own self. Lee Stoller represented everything that she was not. He was her complete opposite.

She excused herself in the middle of a waltz, left him alone on the floor, and found Suzie.

"He is absolutely too much!" she informed her girl friend. "I've never seen anyone quite like him before."

Undaunted by her absence, Lee continued to skate, putting on a one-man floor show . . . until Darrell, the mutual friend who had introduced them, collared him and got him into the seclusion of the restroom.

"Listen, man, you'd better straighten up if you want to take Ellie home tonight. She thinks you're cocky and conceited."

Lee was momentarily deflated, but he quickly retorted: "Hey, I could care less what she thinks. I can pick up someone else out there anytime I want. I will, in fact! There are plenty of girls out there. Let her go home with those two brothers of hers who tagged along. Whoever heard of a 17-year-old girl being chaperoned by her kid brothers, anyway?"

"It's up to you, buddy." But Darrell wanted this match to work out, so he added: "'Course you said awhile ago that you liked her, that she was a good-looking girl."

"Yeah . . . Sure she is. But, man, she's too strait-laced. Yeah . . . I think you set me up for this whole thing just so you could be with her friend Suzie."

Darrell gave up. "Well, make up your mind. She's definitely not the type of girl you're used to dating. But it's up to you."

Lee returned to the floor, but now he was angry. As his anger grew, his acrobatics increased. Skating alone, he was putting on even more of a show.

Meanwhile, Ellie was gliding around the rink slowly, her brothers close beside her. Whenever Lee looked her way—and he did frequently—he presumed that she was pretending not to be watching him.

Then it happened.

Their eyes met.

She really is beautiful, he thought . . . Yeah, she was about the loveliest girl he had ever seen. But . . . He reminded himself of what he had told his older brother Roy just the other day—he intended to remain single. Date, yes. Have affairs with all the women he possibly could. But, play the field. Not settle on any one particular girl. How could just one ever hold his interest?

Still . . .

If he ever did decide to get married—

—Not that he ever intended to, of course—

But if he ever did—

He'd want it to be to a girl like this Ellie Johnston . . .

Lee eased up to her, slowing down to match her pace.

"It's a waltz. May I join you?"

She did not take her eyes off the floor, but she answered softly, "If you like."

He took her small hands in his own. Her fragile fingers touched the callouses of his palm.

"Where do you work?" Ellie asked.

"I'm a fireman on the P & PU," he answered proudly. "But I wouldn't call it 'work.' I just ride around in the engine all day and make sure we don't run into another train."

"I'm a clerk at Bergner's Department Store in downtown Peoria," Ellie said. "And my brother Wayne works at the P & PU."

Lee grinned. "Do you make good money?"

She blustered at his forwardness. "Not bad! It's enough to buy my clothes. I've got a weakness for clothes. I like pretty new things. And I can help out at home. Pay my board. I've got lots of brothers and sisters, and Mom needs the help."

Lee leaned closer as they continued around the rink. Darrell had been right about her not being like the others he dated. Her air of sweet innocence was doing something to him that he wasn't sure he was going to like.

Yeah . . .

He even apologized:

"Ellie, I'm sorry if I seemed to be ignoring you earlier. These girls around the rink are just friends.

I've known them a long time. You don't have to worry. If you weren't more important to me than they are right now, I wouldn't be here."

She stayed silent, her eyes still cast downward, her hands tightening their grip on Lee's.

"If you'll give me a chance, I'll prove to you I'm a gentleman. You can trust me. Can I take you home tonight?"

She didn't let her face show her thoughts.

But she was thinking that maybe there was another side to Lee Stoller than her first hasty conclusion. She liked what she was hearing now, and there was a smile in her mind if not on her face. He *was* handsome. Surely there was no harm in letting him take her home . . .

She nodded.

Outside, Lee held the car door while the brothers jumped in the back and Ellie slid demurely into the front passenger seat. He drove the six short blocks and parked where she told him. He recognized immediately this section of East Peoria. And he knew now that he and Ellie had something in common:

Poverty.

Born Leland Lester Stoller on November 26, 1937, Lee was one of eight children to Lester and Emma Stoller who rented a 160-acre farm near Eureka, a few miles from Peoria. At least that was where they lived when he was born. Lee's memory of childhood was that they seemed to move just about every year to another farm. He remembered that they raised corn and beans, that they had some livestock—pigs, chicken, a few head of cattle. And a vegetable garden. There should have been plenty of food at least to go around, but no . . . Apparently his parents had been poor managers. He recalled many nights when he had gone to bed hungry . . . Yeah. Poverty was a familiar sight to Lee . . .

Ellie's brothers, Charlie and Donnie, thanked him politely for the lift, got out of the car, and went inside. He and Ellie were alone. For the first time. Lee sighed with relief and turned to her.

"I come from a large family myself," he said. "There's eight of us kids. I guess I'm the closest to Roy. He and I used to really hang out a lot together." She was listening attentively, not interrupting, so he continued: "I can remember back in the fourth grade Roy and I could tie a thousand bales of hay between the two of us. Do you like music, Ellie?"

Ellie thought it weird the way he changed subjects without a break in the conversation. "Yes," she answered shyly. "I especially like to listen to the 'Hit Parade.'"

For her it was a long sentence. It seemed to her it came out a little stilted . . . like, maybe she was reading from a book . . . and she was uncomfortable about that.

But she was even more uncomfortable parked in front of the house like this. Parked anywhere for

that matter. And she was acutely aware of Lee
. . . so close to her . . . What if—

"That's a radio show, isn't it?" he asked. Then,
without waiting for her answer, he plunged on.
"When I was a kid we never had a radio. Roy and I
used to go sit beneath a neighbor lady's window and
listen to 'The Lone Ranger' and 'The Fat Man.' She
was nice about it. She knew we were out there and
would turn up the radio extra loud so we could hear.
You know what I really liked as a kid, though, Ellie?
Riding around on that old John Deere tractor with
my dad. I thought that was the greatest thing, sitting
up there next to him and watching those big wheels
grind into that dirt." He shook his head, and there
was a faraway note in his voice . . . as though he were
watching a scene from the past . . . "I loved my dad.
I've always felt that he wasn't very happy. He was a
smart man, though. He could have done all sorts of
things with his abilities. But I guess after he married
Mama . . . and all the kids came along . . ." His voice
trailed off, and when it came back he was speaking
more to himself than to Ellie: "Maybe that's why he
drinks so much . . ." Unconsciously he grew intimate . . . as though he were sharing the innermost
part of his life with her . . . "I remember . . . as a kid
. . . Dad would take me down to the tavern, and I'd sit
there on the mahogany counter munching on a
candy bar . . . Dad would disappear after a beer or
two . . . He'd come back . . . with some fancy lady
who smelled of sweet perfume . . . who'd pinch my

cheeks and hemhaw over me something fierce. I didn't like that part. While he was gone, though . . . I didn't know what was going on and didn't care, I guess. The bartender would keep an eye on me while Dad was gone with the woman, and he'd let me play with the jukebox, so I didn't care what Dad was doing. Wouldn't have made any difference, anyway. I was having too much fun punching all those buttons on the jukebox."

Ellie laughed with him, not so much for what he said but because she was beginning to like this brash, honest young man. It was starting to appear that they did have something in common after all. Poverty and drinking fathers for starters. He was a talker for sure.

He was at it again:

". . . But then, when I was 12, I moved out of the house. I went to work for Tub and Emily Lowery, neighbors of ours. They had three children of their own, but they needed an extra hand to help out with the farm chores. You see, Ellie, even at twelve years old I knew I wanted something better for myself than that old farm had to offer. I'd watch Dad come home drunk, he and Mom fuss, Dad abusing her. I knew he was under pressure with so many mouths to feed, so I figured with me gone it would make it easier on him. He and Mom didn't stop me. I don't think they even missed me. Anyway, Tub and his wife were real nice. Treated me like one of their own. The only thing was they couldn't afford to pay me the fifteen dollars a week we'd agreed on, so I had to find work in town. Between going to school, working 'til midnight at the bowling alley, then walking the five miles back to the Lowery farm, I couldn't keep up the pace. I remember the day the principal called me into his office. He told me I had missed 60 days in my sophomore year and asked me how many I planned to miss the next, asking if I might be trying for 75. Then he forced me to make a choice between school and work. I didn't see that I really had a choice. I had to work. So I quit school. Then, at 16, I got my folks to sign the papers and moved to Chicago and went to work for the Santa Fe Railroad as a painter. I made good money up there, a-dollar-ninety-one an hour. When I'd come home on weekends, Mary Sopher and her two boys, Roger and Larry, would meet me in Chillicothe. She was like a mother. My main goal is to be financially well off by age 40."

Lee was holding her hand now. He felt a new experience flow through him, something beyond physical emotion, beyond fleeting desire.

Ellie did not pull her hand away. She felt the trust he had promised earlier. He spoke with such conviction in his voice that she was certain he would do all he said, that he would eventually become what he wanted to be. Yes, he was a talker—but he made sense. He talked on, and she answered him, talking more freely now than she'd ever done with anyone since she was a child. They had the common bond of remembered poverty, and there was magic in sharing with each other the dreams of what poor people could accomplish. But, in addition, he seemed mature. And he apparently had seen so many things and places. Things and places that she had only been able to find in books.

Lee told her of his first love, how the girl's parents had kept them apart. He told her about his tour of duty with the Corps . . . of his duties at the railroad where he now worked . . . that he was staying with Emily Lowery, who was like a mama to him . . .

The front door of the Johnston house opened. Ellie's father appeared in the doorway after turning on the porch light. "Ellie!" he yelled, "it's eleven-thirty."

Where had the time gone? She turned to Lee, sorry that the evening had come to an end. "I better go in. I really had a nice time, though."

Lee reached for her. "Ellie," he blurted, "I think a lot of you. I never thought I'd be saying this to any girl—and maybe I'm coming on too fast for the first date—but could I see you on a steady basis?"

Ellie caught her breath, avoiding Lee's eyes, afraid her own would betray her emotions. Lee began to speak—with authority and confidence now, each word coming out as though he were addressing a large assembly, with total command of himself as well as the elements around him. It was an attitude new to Ellie, and now she was certain the statement she had made to Suzie at the rink was correct: She had certainly never met anyone quite like Leland Stoller . . .

"I promise I won't date another girl." There was a quick break in his voice . . . as though his own ears didn't believe what they were hearing—which was true . . . "I don't want to, now that I've met you. I'll prove to you that you can believe in me."

A train rattled by, and Ellie waited until it had passed before answering, trying frantically to gather her thoughts. "Let me think about it. Okay? I care for you, too, but this is all happening so fast."

"Can I see you tomorrow, Ellie? Can I take you to work?"

"I suppose so, but I have to be there at nine on the dot."

The robust figure of her father appeared in the door again. This time he left the door open.

She gave Lee a quick, bashful kiss and was out of the car before he had time to move.

"I'll give you an answer in the morning, Lee. I've got to have more time to think about this . . ."

4

Next morning Lee leaned over as she climbed into the car, and their lips met before either spoke.

"Do we go steady?" he asked . . . unnecessarily . . .

"I thought about it all night," she said, looking down at the pleat she was trying to smooth in her skirt. "I'd like to give it a try . . . if you won't ever knowingly hurt me . . . ever . . ."

So it began, the magic years of lovers. Lee followed the ritual of introduction to her parents. He was quickly accepted by her family. There was one poignant moment when he sat with Andrew at the kitchen table and admired the sketches Andrew had drawn. They were good, these drawings of railyards and factories, the city and homesites. If Andrew had only pursued an art career . . .

It was tragic to waste one's talents, Lee thought, and he looked up quickly at Ellie, a shadow in his eyes. What if he and Ellie—

But it was not a somber time. They dated every night thereafter. Drive-in theaters were one favorite, long drives in the country on weekends another. Neither smoked. Neither drank. Both had seen the problem alcohol created in their own families—and the much more serious problems in other families. And most of the time they were oblivious of the people around them, being too absorbed in their own company. The time they spent together always seemed to end much too soon. Each moment apart was an eternity. They were falling deeper and deeper in love.

Oddly, there was one small change during this summer that passed so fast—Lee introduced Ellie to country music. Ellie had always been a fan of pop music, but Lee, who kept the radio on in the car, moving or parked, was out to change all that. Country music, he told her, was the backbone of the nation, the American way. His metaphors, mixed with his enthusiasm, were contagious— soon she was familiar with Eddie Arnold, Jim Reeves, and Marty Robbins. She even eventually realized that Faron Young was Faron Young and not what she thought the deejays were saying: "Fair and young . . ." (Wisely she delayed telling Lee of her mistake . . .)

They had dated only six weeks when they announced to their parents that they intended to get married. Both families were enthusiastic.

Ellie had said that she wanted a long and proper engagement. "This marriage is going to last a lifetime, Lee. I don't like divorces. This is the only wedding I will ever have, and I want it to be right. And I'd like a church wedding, too."

"Fine with me. How soon?"

When she said "June, next year," he couldn't believe his ears but he loved her too much not to do as she wished. He reluctantly agreed.

In late spring they moved the date up to the next Christmas. By early summer it was moved forward again, now to August 1. The year was 1959.

It was not until the day of the wedding that the shock came.

At the church.

Minutes before the ceremony.

Deliriously happy, dressed in the traditional white, Ellie was alone in the small room near the altar. Thoughts and dreams of the future danced in her mind, and she turned to the window to look out—

And saw Lee leaving.

His pink and gray Chevy was parked out in front, and he was walking fast, very fast, almost running toward it. As she watched, puzzled, he leaped into the car and drove hurriedly away with his best friend Jim Kimball, and Lee's brothers, Harold and Harley.

He was leaving her.

Just as the doll of her childhood had been almost within her grasp . . . just as the moment of glory in the school choir had been almost hers . . . this greater moment was being taken from her. The preacher of long ago was right; she was doomed . . .

At this bleakest of moments her sister, Carol,

entered, smiling. "Lee forgot the ring, Ellie. Can you believe it? He was standing there talking to the minister when they asked about the ring. He was absolutely stunned and told them he'd forgotten it. He just left to go home and get it."

"Are you sure, Carol? Are you really sure? He's not leaving me, is he?"

Carol laughed, realizing what her sister had thought. "Of course not, honey! He'll be back in a few minutes."

But Ellie continued to stare out the window. It was not until the familiar pink and grey car pulled around the corner that a smile touched her face.

He had come back . . .

The ceremony was beautiful—as Ellie had thought it would be. Then there were the congratulations. And the picture-taking. All the things that went with a wedding.

Meanwhile, outside, brothers and sisters were busy in the parking lot. Cans and other paraphernalia—anything gaudy, anything that made noise —were being attached to the Chevy. Plans were also being made to follow the after-ceremony of "shivareeing" the newlyweds that evening—keeping them awake all night.

Ellie and Lee said their goodbyes and went to the car. Lee had gotten wind of the "shivaree" plans, so the stop at the apartment (three rooms converted from a garage, renting at $60 a month) was just long

In November, having managed to save a little money, they started shopping for a house. Roaches were not the deciding factor. Both wanted a place they could call their home. They finally decided on another converted garage on a small lot at 2206 North Linsley in Peoria. Lee paid $500 down, and they signed the contract for $50 a month on a 7 percent mortgage. The purchase price for the garage was a whopping $5,400—an awfully huge financial mountain, the newlyweds thought. But the lot, 55 × 150, would be large enough for their kids—if and when they came. It was a one-bedroom structure of cement blocks, painted green. Nothing fancy, but—they both agreed—theirs.

They hadn't been there long before Ellie discovered she was pregnant. Lee suggested she quit work, but before she could Lee was temporarily laid off—and Christmas was just around the corner. Her income needed, she stayed at work.

Lee soon found a job with the Colonial Bakery. That meant getting up at 4 A.M. so he could start out in the truck on the bread route. Ellie rose with him, sleepily prepared his breakfast, and then got ready to catch the bus to her own job at Bergner's. She earned nearly $100 a week, and Lee's new position paid about $200. They were able to save nearly a third of their income each week. Since both had known the heartache of poverty they guarded closely against it ever coming again to them.

Halloween, the last day of October, 1960, the

baby was born. Named Tammy Lee after her father, she was "the most beautiful baby in the world." When, a few weeks later, Ellie returned to work, Rose, the wife of Lee's brother Roy, agreed to be the baby-sitter. So each morning Ellie bundled the infant lovingly against the cold of the late fall weather and carried her over to her sister-in-law. Everything went fine for awhile.

And then disaster struck . . .

When Tammy was only six weeks old she contracted pneumonia. At the hospital her parents were forced to stand helplessly outside the glass window that separated them from their child and watch the nurses tend the tiny baby fighting for every breath.

"Oh, Lee! If I could just hold her! She's my baby, and all I can do is just stand here. If I could only hold her!"

Memory of previous times when happiness had been cut off by disaster surged up in Ellie, and it was all she could do to keep from being overcome by fear that something terrible would happen to little Tammy.

She prayed.

Ellie's prayers were combined with tears as she lay sleeplessly in bed at night. Nightmares would torture her when she finally dozed off, nameless fears she could not remember when she woke up crying and Lee tried to comfort her. Lurking in the back of her mind was the old idea that she was unworthy . . . not good enough . . . that Tammy might die because she, Ellie, was doomed . . . the old fears of her childhood rising again to haunt her. She could find comfort in only two things: Lee's love—

And her prayers.

Her prayers were answered. Six weeks later they brought Tammy home, out of danger. And Ellie, five pounds lighter from work and worry, was out of danger, too . . .

(It did not occur to her at the time that she was living out in her own life the everyday trials and triumphs of the country music she would one day sing. She could not see the hand of fate—or destiny —or God—guiding her through the same everyday experiences as those of her future fans.)

Tammy was barely safe at home before Ellie found she was pregnant again. Lee, a proud and doting father, was determined that his child, Tammy, and the one to come would never suffer hunger and humiliation as he had. He now worked even harder, spent longer hours on his bread route. No, his children would never be too embarrassed to eat with the other children at lunchtime, slipping off to eat from a small paper bag carried to school . . . which, some days, contained a half sandwich only, a thin piece of bread wrapped around a smear of mustard or mayonnaise. And, on some particularly hopeless days, nothing in the paper bag at all, the empty sack carried for appearance only. No, it had happened to him; it would not happen to his kids . . . But the fear was like Ellie's own remembered demons and sometimes haunted him.

Like the night Ellie was sewing and Lee watched Tammy playing happily on the floor, her eyes glancing up from time to time with love and trust for her parents.

Lee said vehemently: "Our children will have the very best, Ellie. They'll never want for anything as long as I live. I'm going to be a millionaire by the time I'm 40! They'll have the things you and I never had."

The words of his outburst hung in the room.

Would they come back later to haunt him?

Not at the moment, though. At the rate Lee was going these days Ellie didn't doubt a bit that Lee would make it. He had a natural talent for sales. He approached each customer on his route each day with disciplined enthusiasm. Whether a small county store or a large supermarket, Lee gave his best effort.

But . . .

There is a snake in every Eden, a problem in every opportunity, a balancing factor in every effort.

Yes, sales provided a rewarding career, but sales

could also drain one's emotions, and Lee was now finding himself needing a distraction from the daily routine. He needed what everyone else in the same situation has needed since time immemorial—recreation.

But . . .

With her new job at the Howard Printing Company Ellie had her own problems and could not, at the moment, be expected to be part of that recreation. Lee needed to relieve his pent-up tension. He wanted to go out, to be entertained. He needed action. Ellie came home exhausted. There were still meals to prepare, the children to look after, and the house to clean. Go out dancing? You have got to be kidding! The times Lee asked her she told him she would much rather relax at home with him and the children. Soon he stopped asking. He had said he understood, but most nights now he slumped restlessly onto the couch, his eyes taking on a faraway look.

Any fan of country music would have recognized the situation. Would have guessed what would inevitably come next . . .

The day had been harder than usual for Lee. Driving home, he stopped by a red light. He felt drained and tense, and he was drumming restlessly on the steering wheel, waiting for the light to change when he heard his name called.

"Hi, Lee," she said through the open window of the car. "I missed my bus. Can you give me a lift home?"

"Sure." He recognized Gladys, the wife of Albert, one of his neighbors. "Hop in."

She bounced into the seat, her short skirt sliding up over shapely, nylon-clad legs. They were good-looking legs, and Lee realized he was acutely aware of her presence . . . so aware, in fact, that he began to try to concentrate on the traffic.

Gladys. He remembered her as an attractive girl. The kind that liked to flirt, maybe, because she often seemed to flirt with him when the two couples were together. No big deal, though. He had just assumed that it was part of her nature. Anyway, he was happily married to Ellie and hadn't been thinking of another woman. Besides, Albert was one of his best friends. And it had always been part of Lee's code not to—

"You look like you've had a rough day," she said, brushing the long black hair from her face as the wind whipped it in from the open window. The same wind blew the scent of her perfume into Lee's nostrils.

"Yeah, Gladys. I've been going a-mile-a-minute today."

"I bet you could use a drink. Albert's not home tonight. If you want, stop by my house, and I'll fix you a drink."

Lee didn't tell her that he and Ellie didn't go

for the liquor. On the other hand, the way he felt tonight . . . maybe a drink would—No. Still . . .

"I don't have much time," he said shortly. "But we could stop by the cafe if you like."

She liked . . .

She sat across the table, her eyes never leaving his face. Every time she reached for the ashtray to flick her cigarette her hand touched his arm. A taunting gleam in her eyes matched her voice.

He was getting the message.

"How do you like married life, Lee?"

"Oh, I think it's nice. I really found the right lady."

"You know, I always wanted to date you when you were going with Ellie and I was with Albert. You were a sharp dresser. And always so sure of yourself."

"Well, I can honestly say I've never wanted to date anyone else since I first met Ellie."

"Have you been out on Ellie yet?"

"No. I don't believe in that."

Gladys laughed. She reached over and teased his hair with long, painted fingernails. "You mean you've never really thought about it?"

"I'm a happily married man. I really am."

Gladys lightly brushed her nails against his arm. "I go out on Albert. In fact, we both date."

"You do?"

"Sure. It's an understanding we have. It doesn't bother either one of us. I bet if you're honest with yourself you've thought about going out with another woman. You're just afraid of getting caught. It might get back to Ellie. That's what you're scared of."

"I'm happy with Ellie as my wife. And I respect our marriage."

Gladys put her hand on the back of Lee's neck and teased his hair. "I've heard all the things you did with girls on dates before you married Ellie. Albert told me."

"I was a bit wild, I guess. But that's history." Lee laughed nervously. "I've been trying to change my ways."

"Don't you think I'm appealing, Lee?"

"Gladys, let's talk about something else."

"I've often fantasized about what it would be like to go out with you."

Lee stood up. "We'd better go. I'll be late getting home . . ."

In the darkness of the car, Gladys slipped close to him, her hand resting lightly on his leg, her sultry perfume heavy in the closeness . . . intoxicating him.

"Relax, Lee. I'm not going to bite you. If you're afraid to go to my house, we can go to a motel. You won't regret it."

For one moment he hesitated.

She moved nearer . . .

* * *

When they reached the motel, Gladys went to a pay phone while Lee registered. She said she had to call her baby-sitter and explain she would be a little late. The domestic touch took some of the romance out of the affair. But . . .

They were in the room less than an hour.

And that included the time Lee took for a cold shower afterwards . . .

What Lee didn't know was what was happening at home.

When Lee didn't appear on time, Ellie began to watch the clock. With concern. Lee had never been this late before without calling . . .

Time passed.

The phone rang.

"Ellie, this is Albert."

"Oh, yes. Albert. I thought it would be Lee. He's not home yet."

"I know. And I know why he's not there yet. Do you?"

"What is it? Has Lee been hurt in a wreck?"

Albert laughed. A nasty laugh. "You don't really know your own husband, do you Ellie?"

"What are you talking about? Where is Lee?"

"Lee is at the Capri Motel with my wife."

"Albert! Don't tease me like that! That's an awful thing to say about Lee and about Gladys."

"I'm not teasing, Ellie. Gladys called me on the

way to the room at the motel. She was mad at me and wanted to punish me by going out with Lee."

"I don't believe you."

"Just ask him when he gets home. See what he says. See what he says about—"

Ellie hung up.

When Lee came in the door his smile was strained.

"Where have you been, Lee?"

"Oh, I . . . ah . . . had to work late. Some of those people on the route just wanted to talk and talk."

"Lee, don't lie to me. On top of everything else, don't lie."

"What— What do you mean, baby? I had to work late." *She couldn't know . . . She couldn't possibly know . . .*

"You've been at the Capri Motel with Gladys."

"Oh, no. That's not true," he blurted. "I had to work late. I can verify it by my customers."

"Albert called me. Gladys telephoned him before you went to that room at the Capri Motel. I know all about it."

Lee's denials froze on his lips before the hurt, accusing eyes. "It's true, Ellie. I'm very ashamed of myself. I would give anything if it had never happened."

"How many other times have there been, Lee? How many other women?"

"Oh, no, Ellie! This is the only time I've ever

done something like this. It was a crazy thing to do, but there have been no other times."

"How can I believe you? You betrayed me. You lied to me. I gave you my love, all my trust. I believed in you and thought you would never hurt me."

"Ellie, I swear this is the only time I have ever done something like this. It will never happen again. You are the only one I love. Please, Ellie, please forgive me."

She looked silently at him. The tender face that had shown him love and devotion was now a mask of pain, and the sight brought tears to Lee's eyes.

He repeated, "Please forgive me."

"Your supper is on the table." She went alone to the bedroom and locked the door behind her.

Lee had no appetite and picked at his food. He timidly knocked on the bedroom door. There was no answer.

With the television turned low, he sank onto the couch. His raw nerves found the healing of sleep . . .

He awoke with a start, realizing someone was standing over him.

Ellie.

With a cold, angry look on her face.

Like a stranger.

Lee tried to smile and opened his mouth to speak. She held up her hand to silence him.

"Lee, I want a divorce."

5

*E*llie, don't say such a thing! Please!"
Lee leaped to his feet. He was instantly awake.

"I'm going to leave you, Lee. I can't live with an unfaithful husband."

"Please don't say that. I know there's no excuse for what I did, but I swear it will never happen again. I love you and our baby. Think about it. Tammy is so young. Don't break us up."

"I can never forgive you. I can never trust you again. How can I believe anything you say anymore?"

"Honey . . . I—" Lee reached out to touch her, but she pulled away.

"Lee, you were everything I wanted in life. I was proud to be married to you. I gave you all my faith, love, and hope. And you betrayed me! It's impossible for me to live with you after this."

"Give me one more chance. I made a mistake, and I admit it. Think about us and our family. Don't do anything rash. At least, think about it first. Promise me that."

She hesitated before speaking. "I have been thinking about it. Especially about the family. I'm ashamed for anyone to know. I won't do anything right this minute, but I don't see how I can ever feel the same way again about you."

"Just give me the opportunity to try and make it up to you, honey. That's all I ask."

She looked at him a long moment and then turned silently and went back to the bedroom. There was the small, clicking sound of the lock being turned.

Lee was alone in the living room, still except for the static on the TV where the station had gone off the air . . .

Since he had been old enough to earn his own money Lee had been self-reliant. He had taken the good times and endured the bad, and—until he had met Ellie—had needed no one except himself.

Now . . .

What have I done to myself? . . . to Ellie? . . .

The answer was somewhere in the shadows of the lonely room . . .

It was a sleepless night for Ellie. When morning came she ignored Lee's gentle taps on the bedroom door and remained in bed until after she heard him leave for work. On her job she moved mechanically, numb from the memory of betrayal.

In the days ahead she was polite—but cold—with Lee, though she tried to act normal in front of the children.

She couldn't talk to her family. She had no friend

to confide in. But there was one salesman at work whom she had known for years. He was a close friend. He often joked with her. He seemed the caring kind. Ellie accepted his invitation to lunch and confided in him.

But . . .

His congenial attitude immediately turned amorous . . .

Disillusioned, from then on Ellie avoided him . . . and anybody else she thought might be like him.

But the tension was building up in her. Sooner or later she knew it would show in her work. So she was not surprised the afternoon her boss called her into his office.

"Ellie, something seems to be bothering you. You're not your usual cheerful self."

She broke into tears, and he came around the desk to hold her comfortingly. Like a torrent her confusion and pain poured out to the older, kindly man.

His words were gentle and soothing:

"Call home and tell them you're working late. I'm going to take you out to dinner tonight and get you straightened out."

She went with him, and the quiet evening was calming. She was grateful. Her boss was a perfect gentleman. She did not think of him as a male at all, only as a trusted confidant.

She accepted several more invitations, finding mental release in the conversations with the older man who made no sexual overtures. It was all innocent. There was one thing, though: she admitted to herself that she did find vengeful pleasure in the hurt look on Lee's face when she came home late. He was silently pained. She almost weakened and went to him. But, *No,* she told herself, *he deserves it* . . .

"What you really need to do," her boss suggested one evening, "is to pay him back."

"How?"

"Have an affair of your own."

"*What?*" Ellie was startled.

"Yes, you ought to pay him back good." His voice was casual, even-toned . . . "You know, I think a lot of you. Always have. You should have an affair with me."

Ellie was too stunned to answer . . .

That night when she got home Lee was reading the paper. He looked up at her with a warm welcoming smile. She went quietly into his arms.

"Lee, I do love you. And no one but you. I want our marriage to work. I'm willing to give it another chance. But I couldn't stand it if something like . . . that . . . ever happened again."

"Oh, Ellie . . ." His face showed visible signs of relief. "I promise you I will never hurt you again."

And, Ellie thought, *I'm not going to give you the chance. Maybe it was partly my fault. Maybe I did push you into another woman's arms by not going out dining*

*and dancing with you when you needed me. I should have
known that becoming a mother doesn't stop a woman from
being a wife . . .*

With the security that Ellie's love had again reas-
sured, Lee plunged himself even harder into his
work. It would take time, he knew, for Ellie to
forgive and forget his infidelity. But he was sure she
would try. And time would help.

Ellie worked, too. But her attention was forced
back to her family with the arrival of their second
child, Cindy, October 15, 1961. Baby Cindy was a
very welcome addition to this family . . . but the
small house was getting smaller.

As the family increased, Ellie's intense concern
spread to each child. After the shock of almost losing Tammy, Ellie realized how much they meant to
her. She pushed all the energies of her tiny body
into serving the ones who meant everything to her.
She cherished the moments she spent alone in the
house with the children, secure in the knowledge
that Lee was at work and would come home to her
soon. Her heart filled with joy.

And . . .

In the stillness of the house she sang.

Lullabies soothed the children to sleep. Current
happy songs brought big-eyed smiles to their rosy
cheeks.

But . . .

She never sang when anyone else was in the

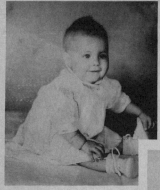

Cristy Lane at five months. Cristy was born on January 8th, Elvis' birthday.

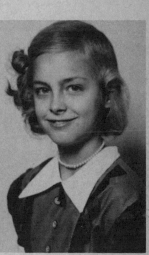

Cristy at ten.

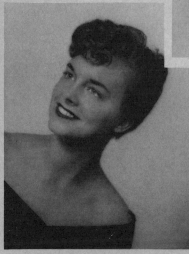

Cristy's graduation picture from East Peoria High School.

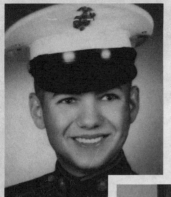

Leland L. Stoller, U.S.M.C.
Born on November 26,
1937, this picture was taken
when Lee was eighteen
years old.

Cristy and Lee's
wedding picture,
taken August 1, 1959.
Left to right: Andrew
Johnston, Pansy,
Cristy, Lee, Emma
and Lester Stoller at
St. John's Lutheran
church, Bartonville,
Illinois.

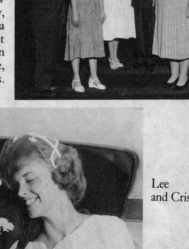

Lee
and Cristy.

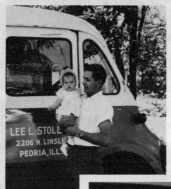

Lee and daughter Tammy.

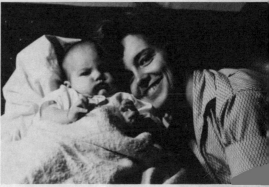

Cristy and Tammy.

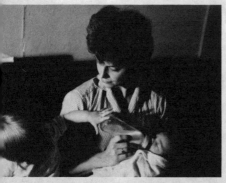

Cristy holding Cindy and
Tammy helping.

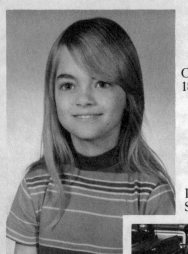

Cynthia Stoller at nine years,
1815 North Otley Road, Peoria.

Lee, Cindy, and Tammy at the
St. Louis Zoo.

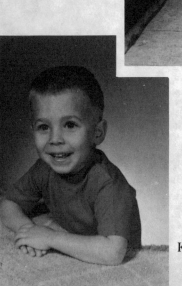

Kevin at four years.

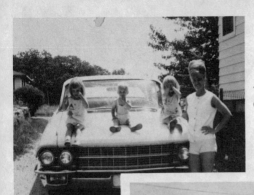

Tammy, Kevin, Cindy, and Cristy.

Cristy and Lee.

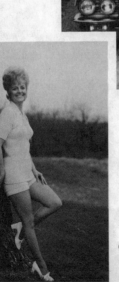

Cristy Lane.

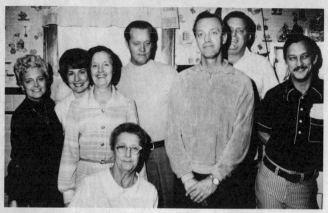

Left to right: Cristy, Carol, Marion, Christy's mother Pansy, seated, Raymond, Ross, Perry, and Donald. Part of Cristy's family of twelve children at Christmas.

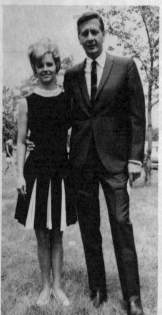

Cristy and Chris Lane.

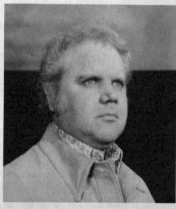

Bobby Mack—the first band that Cristy sang with and one of the best singers around.

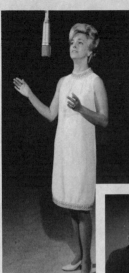

Cristy at Jerry Milam Studio
—her first session.

Cristy's band at Cristy's Inc.
Fred Newell, Ken Hirth,
Cristy, Quentin Good, Jr.,
Mike Shannon.

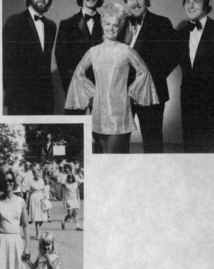

Cristy, Tammy,
and Cindy in St. Louis.

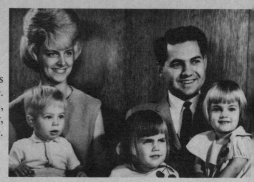

Cristy and Lee's
first family picture.
Kevin, age two,
Tammy, age four,
and Cindy, age three.

Cristy with first band.
Left to right:
Don Edwards—piano,
Jack Allison—lead guitar,
Dave Dringenberg—bass,
Joe Frakes—drums.

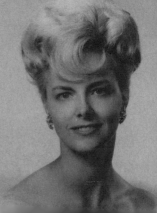

The first picture of
Cristy Lane as a blonde.

house, not even Lee. The buried childhood memories were too strong.

The strain of building and caring for a family and future was taking a toll on Ellie. But not on Lee. He thrived on work. The more he labored, the longer the hours he toiled, the better he felt. It was like developing muscles—the more he used his resources and pushed them to their limits, the greater was his stamina, and the more work he could handle. Besides, he had a goal. He wanted a future for his family. And he had a vow—never to be poor again.

Lee was like that. He thrived on change. He needed a challenge. The P & PU Railroad had offered a steady, comfortable paycheck and a secure retirement. But it was a routine job, and he had become bored.

The Colonial Bakery held more challenge. He was dealing with people, which he enjoyed doing. And he had an incentive: however slight, he did get a percentage from each loaf of bread he sold to a store.

Lee liked selling. He knew he had a gift for it. During the brief time after he got out of the service he had sold insurance for American Republic and had placed in the top 50 salesmen in the country within six months. He might have stayed with it. But there was the pain of the cold Midwest winds whipping down the flat streets, the stinging sleet, the snow, so the softer railroad job further south had looked better. Now, though, going from the railroad to Colonial Bakery had placed him in his natural element of sales. He liked the daily contact with his customers.

But—

He realized that he was reaching the summit of his trade as a bread route salesman. The next step up was a desk job, and that didn't interest him.

So . . .

Somehow Ellie wasn't surprised the day that Lee came bouncing into the house with the news that he had purchased a distributorship from Pepperidge Farms. It had cost him $7,500—but now he was his own boss!

He had purchased the franchise, he told Ellie happily, from Gene Campbell with a few dollars down and monthly payments. It included a large panel bread truck which Lee thought was worth the amount he had paid for the franchise alone. The route served all types of stores, from corner markets to chain groceries. It covered part of Peoria, Bartonville, East Peoria, and Pekin.

On the route, Lee began taking Ellie's brothers Donnie and Charlie along with him to help load and unload the cellophane-wrapped bread and cake kept warm by a gas heater unit in the rear of the truck. And he never tired of his new adventure. It was exciting.

"Ellie," he had declared the first evening, "this is

really it. It's the greatest! Did you know that Pepperidge Bread was started in Connecticut by a housewife who wasn't satisfied with the bread she was getting from the store? She decided that the store-bought bread wasn't good enough nutritionally for her family, so she started to bake her own. Soon all the neighbors heard about how good it was, and they wanted to buy some. Once word got around, she was baking eight to ten hours a day— until finally she had to open more kitchens. Now it's nationwide."

Ellie was back at work. Her income, plus Lee's $200-a-week average from his Pepperidge franchise, enabled them to increase the savings account they had started—and to begin packing. There was a new house on North Otley Road they were looking at, and there was a good chance they might get it. With their third child on the way there just wasn't enough room where they were.

Then Lee changed jobs. As much as he liked being his own boss with Pepperidge Bread, he could hardly turn down the chance to be a field manager for Fuller Brush Company at $20,000 a year. He would recruit and train sales agents. The deal looked good to him, so he took the job. Now they were financially able for Ellie to extend her leave of absence from the job at the printing company while she prepared for the move . . . and for her new baby.

Everything was going fine.
Which meant . . .

The phone rang in the late afternoon, and Ellie, seven months along but feeling more like nine months, groaned as she got up to answer it.

"Ellie, this is Ross." She had recognized her brother's voice, but he sounded a little strange. "Now, Ellie, I don't want you to get upset, but I have some bad news."

"Ross, what is it?"

"Dad is dead. He came home from work and walked into the kitchen and fell down. Mom thought he'd fainted, but he had a heart attack. He died instantly."

Ellie could hardly speak. A shudder ran through her, and she felt very sick. There was a sharp pain in her abdomen, and she knew she had better get to the doctor. Fast.

The shock of hearing about her father's death had caused the baby to drop into the birth canal, and the doctor wanted to put her into the hospital then and there. But Ellie wanted desperately to be with her mother. That was not possible; the best she could do was attend the funeral services. She refused the hospital stay, but she did promise the doctor to stay off her feet.

The burial day Ellie stood next to her mom as the eulogy was given. She had loved her father. He had always been the one to encourage her. When she was a child it was his warm smile that had made her feel special. And now he was gone.

Kevin Leland, their third child, was born May 9, 1963. Now, with three children, Lee worked even harder, and the family prospered. But two years later he switched from Fuller Brush to Watkins Products. Ellie's brothers were baffled by Lee's change since it involved a cut in pay—though with an expense account and furnished company car that Lee said would compensate.

"When is Lee going to settle down?" Perry asked her. "It's just not stable to go from one job to another like that."

Ellie laughed. "Lee knows what he's doing. We've never gone hungry yet."

Up to this point in their lives he certainly had not found anything he couldn't do, she thought. And . . .

That made her feel inferior.

But one warm summer afternoon, as Ellie stood over the sink peeling carrots for dinner, the world changed for her. Fate, destiny, providence, or . . . God . . . tilted her back in the direction she was intended to go.

What a beautiful day it is! she thought as she looked out the window. The children were playing in the yard. Lee was in the living room watching the Yankees and Dodgers battle it out for the 1965 World Series. Suddenly he shouted, cheering his favorite Yankees along.

Hearing him, Ellie smiled. It was good to have him home.

Idly, she began to sing . . .

"Honey, who was that singing on the radio?" Lee asked when he came into the kitchen to get another soda. "I didn't recognize the voice, but I sure liked it."

He was reaching for the handle of the refrigerator. He stopped. He turned slowly toward Ellie. He had just remembered:

There was no radio in the kitchen!

Ellie's face turned crimson. She hadn't even realized that she had been singing. It was just something that came naturally when she was happy and alone. It had not occurred to her that Lee would hear her from the other room.

"Was that you?" Lee stared at his wife in disbelief.

Ellie tried to avoid his eyes, but she nodded.

"Why, baby, I had no idea you could sing! You have a beautiful voice. Sing some more."

"Lee, I sing for myself when I put the kids to bed. That's all. Now, if you don't hurry, you'll miss the rest of the ball game."

"Forget that!" Lee ordered, sounding like the Marine he had been. "I want to hear you sing." He saw that she was embarrassed, understood, and his voice became gentle. "Please. Just one song. Look, I'll even turn my back if that will make it easier."

"Well . . ." Ellie sighed. "Knowing you, I won't get a minute's rest until I do . . ."

She sang "The Tennessee Waltz." Lee stood very still. He could not believe that this was his wife, the shy, sweet little girl he had married five years ago. She had a voice unlike any other he had ever heard. It was honest and pure. Its clarity and simplicity moved him. For the first time in his life he experienced goose bumps listening to a singer. He wanted to hear more.

Reluctantly, Ellie sang for her husband.

And as she sang, there was first the emotional release. That night long ago when a shy young girl in a red polka dot dress had been humiliated and hurt to the soul came back to her . . . But this time—

She stood in the sunlit kitchen singing softly, pretending she was all alone . . . as she had been behind the curtains of the church . . . But slowly there came a change. The little girl who had sworn never to sing again was no longer alone.

She was singing for Lee . . . and the silent music of a beautiful world accompanied every word . . .

6

*E*llie felt silly standing in front of a chair with a microphone taped to it. (She had been too nervous to hold the mike in her hands, so Lee had taped it to the chair.)

How did I ever let Lee talk me into this?

One minute she had been singing in the kitchen, the next here she was out in her living room singing on tape. She had tried to explain to Lee that she didn't want anyone else to hear her sing, but he had insisted. So here she was singing along with one of her Patti Page albums while Lee turned the volume down just low enough so that her own voice would be recorded on tape.

She smiled at her captive audience now quietly sitting on the floor around her. Tammy, Cindy, and Kevin were fascinated at the prospect of hearing their mom's voice come through a machine, and they were very careful not to make a sound.

Lee played the tape back.

"That's great, honey. You sound just like a professional."

"Lee, you're being ridiculous!"

"I don't think so. Well, I might be prejudiced a little, but I know how to take care of that. We'll get an outsider's opinion."

"I am not going to sing for anyone, Lee. So, please, let's drop this."

"Now don't you worry, honey. I will take care of everything."

Ellie was sure that Lee's obsession with her voice would die out in time—until he brought home Bobby Mack, Peoria's most popular night club singer. He explained: "You know those tapes we made in the living room? I had them transferred to a cassette, and I've been carrying it around with my little recorder in the front seat of the car just waiting until I ran into Bobby so I could play them for him."

"Right there in front of the dry cleaners!" Bobby said with a chuckle. "Lee sat that little recorder on the hood of his car, and you should have seen the people gather around to listen."

By now Ellie was blushing visibly.

"You have a wonderful voice, Ellie," Bobby said. "Even through the little cassette speaker I could tell you can really sing."

She laughed nervously and mumbled, "Thank you." She was so embarrassed! *Lee and his projects . . .*

"She doesn't think much of her talent," Lee explained to Bobby. "How can I get her started? Convince her how good she really is?"

Bobby smiled broadly. "Best way in the world—bring her by the club and see what the public thinks. That's what counts. All the critics and experts in the world don't mean a thing if the public doesn't like you."

"I think she's great!" Lee declared.

"I do, too. Would you sing for me now, Ellie?"

Ellie looked at Lee. She couldn't possibly sing for this man who was practically a stranger. Why, she still couldn't even look at Lee and sing at the same time!

"Just one song, honey," Lee implored.

"Lee, please!"

Bobby noticed the tension. "No problem. It's a lot different singing here than in front of people in a club. I would feel real foolish myself if some stranger walked into my house and said, 'Sing!' Why don't you two come by Wayne's Club tonight? I'll call Ellie up to sing a few songs, and we'll see what the fans think."

Ellie couldn't believe it when Lee agreed. She had no intention of getting up on a stage and singing for anyone. But it all happened so fast she didn't have a chance to object until after Bobby left.

"Lee!" she said angrily, "why did you say we would go when you know I'm not going to do it?"

"Oh, honey, don't be afraid." Lee chuckled softly. "Have confidence in yourself. I do."

"I could never get up and sing for a group of people, Lee. I told you that when you started this whole business."

"Ellie—"

"Please, Lee."

"Okay. I won't force you to do anything. But let's just go to the club tonight and get the feel of things. I don't want to hurt Bobby's feelings after he invited us."

"Well . . . I wouldn't mind going to the club. But not to sing!"

"If you get there and want to sing, fine. Otherwise, you don't have to."

"Promise?"

"I promise." Lee kissed her. "Now, why don't you go upstairs and pick out something pretty to wear for tonight."

They arrived at the club fairly early, but already it was crowded. Wayne's Club had a warm atmosphere, cozy tables, soft amber lighting. The crowd tended to make Ellie nervous, but the comforting atmosphere counteracted that. Except that Bobby came over. "Hi!" he said cheerfully. "Sure am glad you could make it. All ready to sing for us tonight?"

"Oh, I don't think I'm going to sing, Bobby," Ellie said, looking around her at all the strange faces.

"Well, you don't have to if you don't want to. But if you change your mind, I'll need to know your key. Lee says 'Paper Roses' is one you like. Hum a little of it for me."

Ellie tried to hide the tremor in her voice as she sang—singing so softly that Bobby had to lean over intently. But she didn't want anyone at the nearby tables to overhear.

"Okay. I think I got it." Bobby straightened up. "Well, I have to get back to work. Enjoy yourselves, kids."

Ellie and Lee danced every number. Ellie was light on her feet. She loved it when Lee took her in his arms to dance slow. She felt safe and happy. She rested her cheek against his. She had completely forgotten about singing.

It was late in the evening when they sat down to enjoy their drinks. Lee was just getting ready to order Ellie another Seven-Up when a drum roll came from the stage.

"Okay, friends," Bobby announced. "Everybody having a good time?" There was applause from the audience, and he continued: "Well, good! Because tonight I have a rare treat for you. Earlier today I heard a little housewife sing—a little housewife from right here in Peoria."

Ellie tensed. She looked at Lee, terror in her eyes.

"She has never sung with a band before, and this is the first time she's ever performed in a club. But she has a fantastic voice, and you're going to love her. Let's have a big welcome for Ellie Stoller!"

Ellie sat rooted to her chair. *This can't be happening,* she thought. *I can't go up there and sing!*

The spotlight turned its bright beam in her direction. There was vigorous applause . . . which, oddly, encouraged her. But she cringed, wishing she could disappear. Then Lee was standing and holding out his hand to her. She looked at him pleadingly. The applause grew louder. There was no escape.

Not knowing what else to do, she took Lee's hand. He guided her to the stage. He was beaming with pride as she stood on the bandstand.

Panic gripped her. *What am I doing up here?* she asked herself, staring at the sea of faces in front of her. She was sure that they could all hear her knees knocking. Nausea gnawed at her stomach. Her palms were clammy and cold. She pressed her hands together and took a deep breath.

For an instant Lee wondered if he had pushed her too far too soon. Maybe she really was too afraid to sing . . . But he whispered, "You can do it, Ellie. You can do it!"

The band played the opening bars of "Paper Roses"—and suddenly Ellie was singing. But she was staring at the back of the club, over the heads of the audience, and she was not sure that in her fright she was remembering the words. All she wanted to do was finish the song and get off the stage.

Ellie's voice seemed to have a life of its own. It was full of innocence and emotion. It was different from that usually heard in a night club. The clink of glasses stilled. The idle chatter dwindled . . . then ceased. One by one the audience turned attention to the little lady with the soothing voice. Lee's eyes traveled from Ellie to the audience. He had never been prouder in his life.

When Ellie finished, the audience responded eagerly. "More! More!"

"I don't know another song," she mumbled to Bobby. But the applause would not subside.

Lee said to Bobby, "Play 'Crazy Arms.' She knows that one."

She sang, but when she finished this one she ignored the applause and requests for more and hurried back to the haven of the table and Lee. Dancers stopped by to tell her they liked her singing. People seated nearby leaned over to compliment her. Ellie blushed. Lee beamed.

During the next intermission Bobby came down from the stage. "Ellie, you did a fine job. You have a natural talent. All you need is experience. Please stay with it."

She was too shaken to say anything. She smiled feebly.

Several months later Ellie sat quietly in the car next to Lee as they drove toward Bloomington, 50 miles east of Peoria. She was wishing she had never gone to Wayne's Club that first night. Almost every weekend since, Lee had taken her there to sing—no matter how many times she tried to tell him how difficult it was for her.

And now he was taking her to a different club in

a different city . . . a whole new band . . . a whole new set of faces . . .

"It's just another audience, honey," Lee said, responding to his wife's silent stare. "And, besides, you know the bandleader—Bob Crutcher. Remember? You met him when I was with Fuller Brush. He said his band is really looking forward to having you sing with them. There's nothing to be afraid of."

She tried to explain. "People don't frighten you, Lee. It wouldn't bother you to get up in front of a crowd. But . . . I keep thinking they are going to laugh at me . . . Or that I will make a fool of myself somehow."

"Ellie, you have got to get over that! I don't know where you got the idea that people will laugh at you, make fun of you—that you are not as good as others."

She could have told him . . . a nine-year-old girl staring at a doll . . . the red velvet curtains of the school auditorium and a mean-faced, sharp-nosed teacher . . . The images passed through her mind.

"You're as good as you think you are!" Lee insisted. "And you are good! I've watched the audience and seen their reactions when you sing. Believe me, they love you."

The club was packed. Unusual for a Friday night. To Ellie it was reliving the first night at Wayne's Club all over again. Even though in the past few months she had begun to feel almost comfortable at Wayne's after so many weekends, now all that self-assurance began to vanish here among all these strangers. And what if the band couldn't play her songs the same way Bobby's band did?

She sat at her table sipping a soft drink. Like most night clubs the room smelled of stale alcohol and staler tobacco smoke—worse tonight, it seemed to Ellie, than usual. And the crowd was getting louder and bigger. The bandleader came over to discuss the songs she would sing. She felt her hands growing clammy. Her stomach began turning. The room was closing in on her. She would suffocate if she didn't get out—

"Lee! I'm sick!"

"What's the matter?" Her face was beginning to pale, and he was suddenly concerned.

"I don't know . . . I just don't feel well. Can we go home?"

"Sure, honey. Let me get our coats. And I'll explain to Bob that we have to leave."

Outside the cool night air felt good against her skin. She breathed a sigh of relief and settled back into the car seat, relaxed.

Lee looked at her suspiciously. "You seem fine now." He felt her forehead. "And you don't have a fever. Ellie, are you really sick?"

"I . . . I guess it was just my nerves." Her voice shook slightly. "I get so frightened just thinking about singing in front of all those people."

"Ellie!" Lee stormed. "This is something you are just going to have to get over! I drove 50 miles to get here. Now I have to drive 50 miles back. And you wouldn't even get up to sing two songs for me."

She noticed he had said "for me"—not "for them" . . .

"Please, Lee. Don't be angry."

But he squealed the tires entering the highway, and he pushed the car beyond the speed limit . . . 70 . . . 80 . . . And he continued to rave at her: "This is stupid, Ellie! We drive a hundred miles and then you don't sing. The people out there are your friends. They're not going to hurt you. I just don't understand."

"Lee, please. You don't know what I go through every time I get up in front of an audience. It frightens me so. You may be used to speaking in front of crowds because of your sales meetings and such. But not me. It's hard on me."

"You're just being silly. It's not right to keep that voice of yours locked up inside of you, Ellie. You should share it."

She began to cry . . . softly. He touched her hand.

"Honey, I didn't mean to be so hard on you . . ."

His fingers were warm, yet she felt a sudden chill. Was it the night air . . . or the memory of standing in the wings of the high school auditorium?

* * *

That night, in bed, Lee held her quietly in his arms. She was trembling. He came to his decision. "Ellie, I've been thinking. Maybe you ought to see another doctor."

"What? I'm seeing two already. Both of them gave me nerve pills—which haven't helped much."

"I was thinking about a different kind of doctor —a psychiatrist."

Her body stiffened. "I'm not off my rocker, Lee."

"Honey, I know that. It's just maybe a head doctor could find out what's causing these fears of crowds and audiences . . ."

Lee waited in the outer room while Ellie saw the psychiatrist, a woman doctor who had been recommended by a fellow worker of Lee's. When the session was over, Ellie would not talk until they were clear of the office.

"I don't like that woman doctor." It was one of the few times Lee had ever heard her say she didn't like someone.

"Tell me about it, baby."

"All she wanted to talk about was sex. And my mother and father."

"You don't feel any better about things?"

"No! I feel worse, if anything. That woman was awful. It wasn't any of her business, but I told her we had a good sex life. I also told her that I loved my parents, and that I had never thought about killing myself—or anyone else, for that matter. She just wants to give me more pills. Like the others. I don't want to go back to her, Lee."

"Okay, baby. You and I can probably lick your problem anyway. While I was waiting for you I read an interesting article in one of the magazines. About 'positive thinking.' You know, like in the books Norman Vincent Peale writes."

She was too distraught to argue. "Anything you say, Lee. But we have to stop by the drugstore right now and fill this prescription. This will make three different kinds of pills I'm taking now . . ."

That evening, after the kids were tucked in, they lay on the couch, holding each other closely, the TV off and a Jim Reeves album playing softly. But . . .

It's not the time for it, Lee thought, yet he had no choice. "Baby," he said, "my brother's in trouble. Roy. His business in Arizona has failed. They need some help. They want to come back here, and I was thinking that we could let them have the basement. It's got a kitchen, and we could fix up some rooms. What do you think?"

Ellie agreed quickly, knowing that if it were a member of her family he would do the same.

Roy, Rosalie, and their three children—whose ages matched those of Lee and Ellie's children— soon settled in. At first, Ellie was glad to have the company of her in-laws since Lee's work covered three states and kept him away from home four nights a week. She continued to work, and Rosalie acted as baby-sitter, a very indulgent one who, at first, kept close tabs on the six tots romping around the house. Ellie would come home from her job at Howard Printing each evening to face an active environment.

For awhile, all went well.

Then Rosalie tired of her new duties as mother of six and moved headquarters to the couch and television, neglecting the needs of the children, the cooking, and the cleaning chores. The children ran wild all day, and Ellie came home after a hard day's work faced with meal preparation and housecleaning. Ellie hated to do it, but she would have to talk to Lee about the situation.

Yet, when he came home the next time, he was so happy at being back that she hated to bring up the problem. Besides, she was scheduled to appear with Bobby Mack's band again the following night at Wayne's Club—which was something else she needed to talk to him about. The guest appearances were coming much too often.

She would find, however, that as far as Lee was concerned they hadn't even started yet . . .

7

*E*llie, we need to get you on stage with a big band." Lee brought up the subject one morning at 6 o'clock, before she was really wide-awake. "I think we ought to arrange for you to sing at the Hub."

"What's a Hub?"

"It's a large dance hall in Edelstein, Ill. A club with a 14-piece band." Lee got on the telephone, and before Ellie could object, he had talked Bill Hardesty, bandleader at the Hub, into listening to tapes of Ellie. But there was a hitch. Hardesty would hear the tapes today, and three of them would be with accompaniment, and three a capella.

"What's that?" Ellie asked, still in bed and still half asleep. "What's an a capella?"

"Get out of bed and I'll show you," Lee—who had just learned the meaning of a capella himself in his conversation with Hardesty—said. "It's singing without music."

Minutes later he had Ellie, still in her nightgown, standing in the living room singing into the tape recorder microphone. Two hours later he was ten miles away, at Hardesty's house, playing the tape. Hardesty listened intently. When it ended, he ran it back again. He picked up his trumpet and played along with her voice.

"I'm amazed," he said. "Perfect pitch! She keeps the pitch perfectly and holds the right key throughout all three songs. I've never known that before in a non-professional."

"I don't understand," Lee said.

Hardesty explained. "All music is played or sung in a certain key. A lot of singers will go on or off key, sharp or flat. For a singer—especially one without training—to hold the same key all the way through a song without a musical accompaniment is quite unusual. That's why I wanted to hear her a capella. Another thing—her voice has a clear, distinct quality. No slurs. I like that."

"Do you think she could have a career in music?"

"Definitely! She's good enough for me to issue an invitation for her to come to the Hub and sit in with my band anytime she likes. It would probably be too-little notice for her to be ready, but I could use a female vocalist tonight. My regular singer is sick."

"We'll be there!" Lee exclaimed.

Of course he had not consulted Ellie. When he did, she was shocked, refused, finally relenting . . .

The Hub was filled to capacity, over a thousand people. But the band kicked off the familiar introduction to "Paper Roses," and Ellie grew a little more comfortable. She sang . . .

When she finished the second song, the crowd roared with applause. Ellie, still shaky, walked from the stage.

"You were wonderful!" Bill Hardesty told her during intermission. "And you're welcome to sit in with my group anytime."

The next few months Lee worked even harder to come up with new ways to promote his wife's new career. It wasn't easy. There were stage clothes to buy. They had to pay a baby-sitter when she performed at the clubs. And since Ellie was only a guest singer, there was no pay. The expenses had to come out of their regular budget, and it was trying.

Yet something new and strange was happening. As Lee's constantly examining gaze went from Ellie to the dancers at night, he could feel a rapport building between them. Her voice, sincere and warm, generated a magical bond merging singer and listener. Ellie was no longer just singing; she was now a welcome visitor to the ears, minds, and hearts of the audience. She was winning them over.

But the strain was beginning to show on Ellie. Working at the printing company, keeping house, and taking care of the children took all her normal energy. The added burden of battling stage fright was too much, and she was getting more tense and nervous. Stomachaches began . . .

Then one night Lee called from Madison, Wisconsin, during a break in a sales conference. "Honey, I've got it! You have to write a song."

"Honestly, Lee, you are being ridiculous."

"No, I'm not. I've been reading about all the big stars in the country music magazines, and that is how most of them got their breaks—writing and recording their own songs. You can do the same."

"Lee, I still get nervous just *thinking* about performing. And you want me to write a song!"

He's pushing me too hard and too fast, she thought. But after she hung up the phone, she began pacing the kitchen floor. The children, at the kitchen table, watched her.

"Mommy's mad at Daddy," Tammy announced to her siblings. The three of them watched as Ellie sat at the table and with pencil and paper began to hum and write, hum and write.

"Sing out loud, Mommy," Cindy asked.

"It's a surprise for Daddy . . ."

On Friday evening, after Lee had emptied his suitcase, showered, and joined the family for dinner, Ellie handed him two pages of neatly-written lyrics.

When he read the titles, he smiled broadly. "OK, honey, I get the message." The first song was entitled "Stop Fooling With Me." The second was "Heart in the Sand." Ellie had the melodies in her head, and she sang them for Lee there at the table.

"I told you that you could do it, baby," Lee exclaimed. "We're going to make tapes of these and send them to the biggest people in the music business."

Lee, constantly thinking ahead where Ellie's career was concerned, had kept in contact with Jerry Milam, a young man in Pekin who was trying to get started in the recording business. Jerry had converted two small rooms in the basement of his home into a recording studio. Here, with Bobby Mack's four-piece combo providing the background, Ellie made a two-track tape recording of each song.

"I think you've really got something here," Jerry told Lee. "I'd like to sign Ellie to a recording contract. I'm trying to start my own label, and I'll pay scale. I can't pay you any money right now, but if I get going and sell records, who knows?"

They signed a one-year standard recording contract. No money was exchanged, but Lee did get a dozen tapes of Ellie's songs. The session cost Lee $300. For that he got tapes of the two she had written, also "Four Walls," and her favorite, "Paper Roses."

Watkins Products still supported them, and Lee could not neglect his work, but he sent the tapes to radio stations and singing stars. One went to Marty Robbins in Nashville. Another was sent to the National Barn Dance in Chicago.

Lee was out of town again when Ellie went to the mailbox one morning and casually went through the small stack of letters and bills. Suddenly her eyes widened as she saw the return address on one very official-looking envelope . . . *The National Barn Dance Radio Show.* She swallowed hard. And refused to open the letter. Later that day, when Lee called from Springfield, she told him about it.

"Open it, baby! Right now. Read it to me."

Her heart began to pound as she read the words . . . they liked her voice, and they wanted her on the show. She couldn't believe it.

Lee was ecstatic. One of his dreams was coming true.

That Saturday night came all too soon for Ellie, and she was silent most of the way to Chicago. Even at the receptionist's desk, shaking hands with Dolph Hewitt of the National Barn Dance, she was wary. "I don't know if I can make it through this, Mr. Hewitt."

"You'll do just fine. We get thousands of letters and tapes from people wanting to appear on the National Barn Dance. We only consider the best. You wouldn't be here if we didn't think you were good enough."

She met others on the show . . . Orrel Samuelson . . . Red Blanchard . . . Arkie, the Arkansas Wood-chopper . . . Bob Atcher . . . and Dolph's wife, Ruth, of the Johnson Sisters. *If they go through this ordeal every weekend, maybe I can, too . . .* she thought.

But what happened at rehearsal brought out how

little she knew about music. Dolph, looking at the sheet of paper listing her songs, asked: "What key do you want to do 'Paper Roses' in?"

Ellie looked at him, puzzled. "I don't know my keys." A few of the musicians began to smile. *They're laughing at me! Why did I ever agree to do this?* Again the all-too-familiar feeling of shame and embarrassment flooded over her.

"A key is the range in which a singer sings and the musicians play. If they aren't the same, it sounds awful."

"I thought 'C' was the only key," Ellie said timidly. "In high school choir practice I used to see a 'C' on the music sheet."

Dolph looked puzzled. Then he suddenly smiled in recognition. "The bass clef! It does look like a 'C' turned backwards. Well, no matter. You just start singing, Ellie, and we'll find your key."

She tried desperately to keep the tremor out of her voice. But, as she practiced, every now and then she would look over at Lee, see his beaming face, and say to herself: *I can't let him down. This means too much to him.* So she got through rehearsal.

Later, waiting in the wings for her name to be announced, it was another matter. Just like the high school auditorium . . . She was shaking all over. The pressure was too much. Then her name was called. Ellie did the only thing she had learned to do that would give her strength to step out on the stage. It had never let her down before. Silently she began to pray: *Our Father, Who art in heaven, hallowed be Thy name* . . .

Dolph was saying: "We have a special guest from downstate, from Peoria, tonight. This is a little lady I think you are going to be hearing a lot more from. Tonight she is appearing in her first live professional performance on radio. Making her debut on the National Barn Dance is . . . Ellie Stoller!"

No one in the audience had any idea what the little-girl-like figure on stage had gone through before walking up to that microphone. Not even Lee. All he saw was his pretty little wife in her light blue dress trimmed with red—the dress he had bought for her especially for tonight. Against the bales of hay and the wooden picket fences that decorated the stage, she was a tiny figure, almost a doll . . . vulnerable . . . Yet he thought she had never looked nor sounded better than she did tonight.

Ellie hardly noticed the thunderous applause that followed her as she walked off the stage after her final song. All she wanted was for it to be over. Lee met her in the wings, and she looked at him questioningly.

"You were terrific!" He hugged her tightly. She sighed audibly . . . as though a big weight had been lifted from her shoulders.

Dolph asked her to join him after the show as he signed autographs. To her surprise—and embarrassment—she was asked to sign some herself.

"Ellie, you have a unique style all your own," Dolph said after the last autograph was signed. "You have a soft, appealing voice. Your enunciation is perfect. I hope you'll come back and sing for us again. You do have a future in this business, you know. It's a lot of hard work, but I think it's worth it."

As they were leaving, almost as an afterthought, Dolph said to Lee, "If you're going to pursue a career for Ellie, it would be a good idea to think about a name change. Ellie Stoller is a little hard to remember. You need something catchy."

He handed Lee an envelope which they did not open until they had walked out to the car. Lee held the contents under the dash light. A check for $87. "Ellie, look at this. You got paid for tonight! I was so excited about your getting to sing on the show I didn't even think to ask about that. Why, that's even more than the Grand Ole Opry pays! Honey, maybe we ought to frame this. The first money you ever made singing!"

Lee spent the next couple of weeks looking for a new name for Ellie. And, pepped up by the phone calls he had received praising her performance on the National Barn Dance, he began to think of something else . . . Nashville, Tennessee . . .

"Yeah, I've been to Nashville several times," Bobby Mack, visiting him one afternoon, said. "I even made a record—'Indian Love Call.' It didn't do much, though. You really need a lot of money for promotion—plus a good business sense."

"Nashville is definitely in my plans," Lee said, "but I want to build up Ellie's repertoire of songs first. I don't want to go down there unprepared. Besides, I'm still looking for a stage name for her."

"Have you come up with anything yet?"

" 'Tammy Lee.' But that's too close to Tammy Wynette and Brenda Lee."

"Besides," Ellie added, returning from the kitchen where she had been pouring their colas, "that's my daughter's name."

So the search went on. Ellie and Lee spent hours poring over movie magazines—and even the telephone directory—searching for the right name. For Lee, it was serious business. For Ellie, it was fun—and a way to share the time with the man she loved. As far as she was concerned it wouldn't bother her if she never sang in public again. She was happier singing in the kitchen anyway . . . no one there to judge her or make fun of her . . .

One day Lee stopped at a record store to pick up a Jim Reeves album. When the salesclerk rang up the purchase, she dropped a printed record chart of the top 50 songs, compiled by WJJD radio station in Chicago, into the bag with the album.

At home, Lee put his new purchase on the record player, turned up the volume so that Ellie could hear in the kitchen where she was preparing dinner, dropped on the sofa, took off his shoes, and propped his feet up on the hassock. Thus comfortable and relaxing to the music, he idly glanced over the record chart that Station WJJD had compiled. The names of the station's disc jockeys were printed on one side, and Lee, out of force of habit, ran down the list: . . . Don Chapman . . . Mike Larson . . . Roy Stingley . . . Honest John Trotter . . . Chris Lane—

Chris Lane! Chris Lane! Lee got up slowly, saying the name over and over. He walked into the kitchen and looked at his wife standing over the sink.

"Ellie, I've found your new name."

"What is it?"

"Cristy Lane."

"Cristy Lane? Cristy Lane . . ." She smiled. "I like it!"

Lee kissed her, then held her at arm's length.

"Hello, Cristy Lane!"

8

*H*ow did you happen to come up with it,
Lee?"

"From a radio record chart that the lady
at Jay's Music Store gave me. The disc jockey, Chris
Lane. I took the 'h' out of the first name and added
the ty."

"Lee! You can't do that!" Ellie was shocked.

"What do you mean, I can't do that? I knew it was
right for you the minute I saw it."

"No, taking the man's name. You can't just take
somebody's name like that!"

"Sure I can!" Lee laughed. "People do it all the
time."

"Well, I certainly won't." Ellie was adamant.
"That's like stealing. I won't take his name without
his permission."

"Oh, honey—I mean, Cristy—"

"I mean it, Lee. I'm still Ellie Stoller. I won't be
called Cristy by you or anyone else until you get
permission from Chris Lane."

Lee was more than a little miffed. His little wife
was putting her foot down more and more it
seemed. On the other hand, he *had* been trying to
get her to have more self-confidence . . . He would
have to make the trip to Chicago, like it or not.

* * *

Chris Lane was a neatly-dressed, cordial man in his early thirties. His greeting, over a desk piled high with records, was relaxed and cordial. "What can I do for you, Mr. Stoller?"

"Mr. Lane, I have this little lady who I think is a sensational new singer." He passed her picture across the desk.

"She is cute. What's her name?"

"Cristy Lane," Lee answered, a half-smile on his lips.

"Oh?" It was the disc jockey's turn to smile, and he did so broadly. "This is one tape I've got to hear. 'Cristy Lane,' eh?"

Lee handed him the tape made by Jerry Milam. Chris put it on a portable player behind his desk, leaned back, and listened intently. Lee watched his face, seeking a sign of approval.

When the tape finished, Chris asked, "Is Cristy Lane her real name?"

"No. It's Ellie Stoller. My wife."

"I would like very much to meet my namesake."

"When?"

Chris leaned back, hands behind his head. "I emcee a TV show, 'Swing Around.' "

"I know the show. I understand you have eight million viewers."

"I might be able to give her a shot at it, but I need to see her perform first. Roy Stingley and I take turns as MC at the Rivoli Club here in Chicago. I would like to have my namesake sing a few numbers at the club this Saturday night—if that's convenient with you."

"We'll be there." Lee shook hands and started for the door. He paused and turned back. "Oh . . . What can I tell her about using your name?"

"Tell her to use it with my blessing. I hope she sells a million records with the name Cristy Lane."

The Rivoli Club, one of the most popular night spots in Chicago, was in an old theater building remodeled to seat over 2,000. Cristy surveyed the multiple layers of tables surrounding the huge stage. *I will be confident,* she told herself as she walked to the microphone. Deliberately, she looked out at the big audience. Beyond the glare of the spotlight that burned into her eyes she saw the faint flicker of the table candles, the dim glow of an occasional cigarette. She felt, rather than saw the two thousand people before her that were watching her every movement, that would be hearing her every inflection of sound.

An odd thing happened.

She began to draw strength from the closeness and kindredship of the listeners, as she sang "Crazy Arms" and "Four Walls" began to feel a sharing of the experience with the thousands. Up to now she had always sung for Lee's approval. He was her critic and her judge. But tonight she began reaching beyond Lee, her voice consciously seeking out the entire audience. A great wave of emotion carried her up, up . . . and the audience with her . . .

The applause was deafening.

"Cristy, you're great!" Chris Lane said. "I want you on my TV show!"

For once she was ready to say "Yes" before being prodded by Lee, and her mouth was open to speak.

But Lee spoke first. "We would love to, Chris. But it will have to wait until we get back from Nashville."

Cristy was dumbfounded.

"From *where*, Lee?"

"From Nashville, honey. Didn't I tell you?"

The way it had come about was that Dolph Hewitt had wanted Cristy back on the National Barn Dance the next Saturday night. He had told Lee he would help put him in touch with the right people in Nashville for a really professional recording of Cristy. And Lee wanted the "Nashville Sound" for his singer-wife.

He wanted something else, too . . .

He wanted to complete her image change—and that involved changing her hair to blonde. It took a lot of persuasion, but finally she agreed. The young children looked at their mother as though she were a stranger.

"What's the matter, Tammy?" Cristy asked. "I'm still the same person. Don't look at me so funny."

"What happened to your hair, Mommy?"

"I just changed the color. Daddy wanted me to. Do you like it?"

"It's pretty. You just look different."

They made the trip to Chicago, and Dolph Hewitt introduced "Cristy Lane" to the radio world. Ellie felt a touch of sadness as she stood receiving the applause. She was the same person as before. Her voice was the same as before. But it was as though a new woman was receiving the credit another had worked for. For 26 years she had been Ellie Stoller, wife, mother, would-be singer. Now Ellie Stoller slipped into oblivion, and Cristy Lane, professional singer, took the stage—for now, and for the future . . .

"I like the name change," Dolph told them in his office after the show. "You're going to be surprised at the difference it makes."

"Does a name matter that much?"

"Sure. Would you go to a movie starring Spangler Arlington Brough?"

Cristy laughed. "Never heard of him."

"You've watched him many times—as Robert Taylor. Most movie stars and singers change their names to one that fits their image."

Dolph had something else to contribute. "Lee, I've called Cliff Parnum in Nashville. He's an old friend. And he's the best in the business. He'll be expecting a call from you."

"What does he do?"

"He's an arranger and a producer. He can take Ellie's song—one she's carrying in her head—and produce a really professional recording from it."

"Can you explain that to Cristy? I still have a lot to learn about the business."

"Sure. An arranger takes a piece of music—say, just a melody as your song is—and 'scores' it. That means he puts the musical notes down on paper. Then he writes a different arrangement for each instrument to get the sound he wants. All the instruments are playing the same music, of course, but the dominance varies according to what the arranger is looking for. Each instrument must complement—support and enhance—each other. And do the same thing for the vocalist. That's not the end of the job, though. The producer takes the score and locates, hires, and puts together the talent to make the recording. He knows what each is capable of doing, and how much to pay them. Cliff is both an arranger and a producer. He has handled such stars as Brenda Lee and Connie Frances. And he is—above all!—honest. That's one reason I recommend Cliff. He shoots straight. He won't take advantage of you. His cost will be reasonable."

In the next few days Lee made several phone calls to Cliff Parnum. He and Cristy took all their money from the savings account, borrowed some more, took time off from work, and headed south for Nashville.

It seemed to Cristy that a lot had happened in a very short time.

I wonder how it will work out . . . she thought . . .

9

Nashville!
Even the sound of the name brought visions of country music. The city itself was like a throbbing heart of sound—fiddles, guitars, banjos. Cristy and Lee checked into the Allen Hotel, had lunch at the hotel restaurant—Martha's Kitchen—and took on the role of typical tourists.

Cristy would have stayed for hours in the Country Music Hall of Fame reliving the careers of Gene Autry, Jimmie Rodgers, Patsy Cline . . . and others. She felt she was becoming a small part of this world, and the thought thrilled her.

Lee was looking at the commercial side. He saw the tidal wave of dollars crashing down on Nashville. Music Row in the downtown area had been reclaimed from the slums by the music czars. Abandoned houses had been torn down to make room for new buildings—or remodeled—to house the industry. The price of land in the area had gone from $1,500 a lot when the project began in the early '60s to $50,000. Now it was the domain of publishers, booking agencies, record companies, and the people who made the records spin on turntables around the world.

The Nashville story was told through the trade publications: "Cashbox," "Record World," "Billboard," and "Music City News."

They met Cliff Parnum. He was casually-dressed and soft-spoken. He looked like a friendly small-town merchant, but his conversation overflowed with knowledge of the music business.

"Dolph and I go back a long way," Cliff said. "If Dolph says this little lady has talent, I believe it. I know how it is to start in this business with all the expenses and problems. I will charge you only my $500 minimum to arrange and produce your tapes. The rest of the cost—musicians, background singers, technicians, and studio rental—will run an additional $3,000."

"Dolph gave me the general idea," Lee said. "He explained that the taping facilities here are superior to what we used before."

"The tape you brought was two-track. We will be

recording on three-track. But first we have to pick out the songs which will be best to record for Cristy."

So Lee, Cristy, and Cliff spent the rest of the afternoon making the selections. Four songs were picked. Cliff liked the two Cristy had written, "Stop Fooling with Me" and "Heart in the Sand." Then they settled on Jeannie Pruett's "Janie Took My Place." The fourth song was "I'm Saving My Kisses."

The next day Cristy and Lee were at Cliff's office early, and Cristy watched what for her was the fascinating spectacle of Cliff writing the melody of her songs down on paper in musical notes. Cristy had sung them from her memory previously, and with musicians who played by ear. Now they were a series of musical notes interspersed on lines across a sheet of music.

But there was more to come. She watched Cliff take the piano sheet and make different scores for the various instruments. He did the same with all four songs. "The instruments will come in high or low," he explained, "as needed to blend in with the songs for the effect I want. The instruments must complement and enhance your voice. I've already lined up the musicians and background singers for tomorrow. They are the finest in the business today. Lloyd Green will play steel guitar, with 'Pig' on the piano. Pig is blind. The Anita Kerr Singers will provide the vocal background."

"I'm scared already," Cristy said.

"Don't be. It's all in a day's work."

"But all these people are professionals—and I'm just an amateur."

"Don't feel that way, Cristy. I've been working with so-called 'professionals' for years, and I know you have the natural talent to sing with any of them."

Lee added, "Cliff, I've been trying to tell her she has no reason to feel inferior about her ability."

"Definitely!" Cliff declared. "And remember we are all here to work *with* you. Everyone is on *your* side."

The next morning Cristy was still extremely nervous. They met Cliff at Columbia Studios where a huge Quonset hut had been converted into a studio. *A far cry from the two rooms in Jerry Milam's basement,* Cristy thought. *I'm scared . . .*

She and Lee were ushered into a large area dominated by a grand piano. Shoulder-high panels separated sections where different groups of instruments and the background singers were stationed. An army of microphones stood like waiting sentinels throughout. Cables spread electronic tentacles across the floor. Violins, guitars, bass drums, and other instruments caught her eye. She saw musicians milling about, nonchalantly sharing trade gossip as they unpacked their instruments.

Cliff introduced her to the group and began passing out sheets of music he had arranged. "I'll be over in the control booth," Lee told her. "That window there with the two engineers in it. Want a Coke or something before we start?"

"I'm too nervous to drink anything. I wish you could stay with me." She clung to his hand.

"You'll be okay, honey."

It wasn't so bad after all. Once they started the first song it was just like singing had always been for her. Cliff had told her and Lee that on this three-track recording one track would carry her voice, the second would emphasize the background singers, and the other one would feature the instruments. But she realized she really didn't have to know all that. All she had to do was sing . . .

They stopped, then started over several times— until Cliff was satisfied with the result. The procedure was repeated with each of the other three songs. Then she went to the booth and watched the engineers play back the tapes and blend the sounds.

Fascinated, Cristy watched the veteran hands spin dials and push levers to raise, lower, and mold the sounds from the three tracks. Her voice filled the now-empty studio as the engineers manipulated the background voices and music . . . until her own voice was riding a beautifully-flowing river of sound. Touched emotionally, she reached for Lee . . . to share the moment . . .

*   *   *

She waited at the hotel while Lee made the rounds of the recording companies with the tapes. She was still feeling the glow of triumph. She could not know that Lee was tasting defeat . . .

No doors would open for an "unknown name." The men he asked to see were ". . . in conference," or, ". . . out for the day . . ." If Lee had not been a salesman, accustomed to doors being slammed in his face, he might have quit. But not Lee.

He was able to see Owen Bradley at Decca Records, Chet Atkins at RCA, and Roy Dea at Mercury. But he got only one definite offer—from K-Ark Records. They were impressed and wanted to sign Cristy, but Lee wanted a contract with a major label and turned K-Ark down.

Three days went by.

"It seems no one is interested in Cristy Lane the singer," Cristy said in discouragement.

"Be patient, honey. The right door will open."

But she knew better. "We've spent too much money already—on the trip, making the tapes. We don't have anything to show for it. No contract. Nothing."

"It just takes time. Don't be discouraged. I already have my next step planned. I'll do it from home."

When they returned to Peoria, Lee began a mail campaign, sending copies of the tape, a cover letter, and a picture of Cristy to selected record executives.

Marty Robbins answered promptly, saying he liked the tape and wanted Cristy to come to Nashville to meet him, a thrill for Cristy since Marty Robbins was one of her favorites.

In Nashville, Cristy caught her breath when she saw Marty coming down the stairs into the reception room to meet them. He really did look like his hit song, "El Paso" . . . brightly-polished, high-heeled Western boots, Levis, Western shirt . . . But she was not prepared for his broad, friendly smile.

"Come sit next to me at the piano, Cristy. I want to see if you sound as good in person as you do on the tape."

By now, when she sang, she was aware of the quality of her voice. Clear and melodious, it brought an approving smile to Marty's face. "I like what I hear—very much!" he said after she finished "Stop Fooling with Me" and "Janie Took My Place." "I would like to sign you to a recording contract."

Lee answered for her, "That would be great!"

"There's only one problem. I have let my recording company become dormant, and it will be about six months before I can reactivate it. If you can wait that long, I think we can make some fine records together."

Cristy looked expectantly at Lee. She knew she liked the prospect of singing for Marty's label. And as far as six months was concerned, well, most women can wait patiently for a goal . . .

Lee said, "We're really honored, Marty. But I want to get Cristy's records out sooner."

Cristy's smile faded . . . but she said nothing . . .

"I can understand," Marty said. "I think Cristy will make it big, and I hope you have great success. One word of caution, though. There are a lot of unscrupulous merchants in this business, Lee. Be careful of who you deal with."

"Everybody speaks highly of you, Marty. Could you tell us some of the ones to be careful of?"

"I don't really like to put anyone down. I think you are sharp enough, Lee, to recognize the ones out to take you."

When they left, Cristy expressed disappointment. "Lee! You are so impatient! You want everything right now. Can't you ever wait for something?"

"Honey, six months is a long time in the music business. In that length of time I want to have you 'Number One' on the record charts. We're going to see Johnny Capps while we are in town. He's the head of K-Ark Records. Rather than wait six months, I'm going to pay K-Ark to issue a release for you."

She did not understand.

"Subsidy," Lee explained. "We pay K-Ark to manufacture records from two of the masters we cut with Cliff Parnum. K-Ark distributes, providing promotional material. And I'll work with them on the promotion."

"We don't get paid anything? We have to *pay them*, instead?"

"It's promotion, honey. Exposure. It's an investment—and it will pay off."

Cristy did not answer him . . .

Lee signed the recording contract with K-Ark and paid them $1,000 to manufacture 800 records. He took 500, and K-Ark agreed to mail out 300 to country music stations across the country. The record, a 45 rpm, carried "Janie Took My Place" on one side, "Stop Fooling with Me" on the other.

But the release never got onto the national sales charts. One station in Muncie, Indiana did report it as number one with their listeners. But the stations in Peoria, following a custom of rarely promoting local talent, neglected it. Yet Lee never displayed any disappointment in front of Cristy, always speaking with praise and optimism. He had sensed that her self-confidence was growing, and he would do nothing to shatter that fragile growth. He kept his own dark moments to himself.

Like the night he had slipped into the kitchen after Cristy was in bed and asleep and spread bills, receipts, and bank books across the kitchen table. In the quiet house, he had totalled the cost . . . And to pay for it, he had used all their hard-won savings . . . and put a second mortgage on their home . . .

But . . .
One Saturday they were driving to the grocery store, the car radio tuned to Spence Morris on station WAAP in Peoria.

"Hey, listen!" Lee turned up the volume.

". . . a little lady from right here in Peoria. The sleeve on the recording says she has 'the sweetest voice this side of heaven,' and calls her the female Jim Reeves. There are some kind words on the record sleeve from Marty Robbins and Dolph Hewitt. They say she's pretty good. Let's give a listen to 'Janie Took My Place,' sung by our very own Cristy Lane."

Cristy looked intently at the dash where the car's radio speaker was. It pleased her to hear her voice being broadcast, but it sounded strange to her . . . not like she thought she sounded.

When the song was over she turned hesitantly to Lee, smiling, but embarrassed, too. "Do I really sound like that? Awful?"

"Don't say that, love. It sounds wonderful. It really is 'the sweetest voice this side of heaven.' "

"Lee!"

"One day that voice will be heard around the world."

10

C risty expected things to return to normal after the trip to Nashville. But "normal" is not always pleasant. And in this case it involved two problems: Rosalie alone—and Rosalie and Roy together.

Lee was back on the road. Cristy was back at work. And Rosalie was back on the couch. The kitchen sink was still usually stacked with dirty dishes, and the mess in the living room was still so bad that Cristy suspected it brought a sigh even from Rosalie.

Cristy guessed she shouldn't be surprised. It had been the same way now for . . . how long? Had it just been a year? It seemed more like five. Cristy knew Roy and Rosalie were trying to get back on their feet, and at first she hadn't minded them being there—particularly with Lee gone so much during the week. But . . .

Now there was a new problem, one that threatened to undermine Cristy's new-found security.

For Cristy had started to read all the positive-thinking self-help books she could find. And the Bible had become her constant companion. She had started reading to the children from the Bible nightly and had added more and more reading from it to herself when she was alone. She had always been quietly religious. Now it was as though she were rediscovering the deep security that comes from God. The self-help and positive-thinking books complemented her Bible reading. They were like other tracks . . . instruments and background singers . . . complementing the Master Track . . .

But Roy and Rosalie seemed to delight in undermining the personal security Cristy was now feeling. The worst point of attack came at night, after all six children were put to bed and Rosalie and Roy came upstairs to watch TV with Cristy.

Roy liked her well enough, Cristy guessed. But for some reason she couldn't explain, it seemed he always resented her marrying his brother. As for Rosalie, there was apparent envy to contend with. Probably because of role reversal. Rosalie in high school had been the queen of everything, and Cristy had been shy and withdrawn. Now Cristy had success—however small—and Rosalie . . . well, the setback had been hard on her. Cristy could understand all this. What she couldn't understand was why Roy and Rosalie turned the conversation every night to a single theme—Lee's sexual activities before he met Cristy.

"He had women chasing him all the time," Roy said.

"Please, Roy, I don't want to hear that kind of talk."

"Well, it's the truth, Ellie." Roy adamantly

refused to call her "Cristy." "There wasn't a woman who wouldn't jump in bed with him."

"Yes," Rosalie added. "He was a real ladies' man. I bet he still is. He has that look about him."

"And, you know," Roy added, "he's not sleeping alone every night. Not as good-looking as he is. I bet he's got a different girl every night."

Variations of these accusations came nightly. And eventually they had an effect on Cristy—probably, she thought, because of the memory of Lee's taking Gladys to the Capri Motel that night. Things got worse. Cristy went from one doctor to another seeking relief from the tension and nervousness building up in her. Each of them prescribed a different tranquilizer. At first she thought the prescriptions helped. Then she found that she had to take more to calm herself, and she needed sleeping pills to get to sleep. Worse still, her efforts to explain the problems to Lee were fruitless.

"They drill at me over and over about your being unfaithful to me, Lee."

"Oh, they're just talking. There's nothing to what they say. You know that."

"I just can't take the pressure much longer, Lee."

"Don't pay any attention to them. Their being here is better than you being alone. I feel better being away on the road when I know they're here with you."

It's no use, she thought. *He won't listen . . .*

And then there came a certain Friday night . . .

* * *

Lee was unusually tired. He had met, trained, and worked with scores of new recruits all week for Watkins Products. He had driven 150 miles to reach home from his last meeting. Nerves frayed, exhausted, his only thought was to relax with his family.

As for Cristy, she had reached the breaking point. No sooner were she and Lee alone in the bedroom than her pent-up emotions burst into tears and words. Between her sobs she told Lee she would no longer stand the hammering she was getting from Roy and Rosalie. And she added, "Please tell me, Lee. You are true to me, aren't you?"

"Oh, Cristy, for heaven's sakes!" he snapped. "I've got no time for this foolishness. I had a bad day, and I'm tired. I have to have some sleep."

"Lee, please talk to me. I have to hear you say you love me."

"Cristy, this is all so stupid! I don't want to hear any more. I'm going to sleep."

Silence from Cristy . . .

Which he did not notice.

When Lee awoke, roused by that feeling some call a premonition, Cristy was not in bed with him. A thin wash of light came from under the bathroom door. Something . . . or Someone . . . pulled Lee toward the silence beyond.

Cristy lay on the floor, a sleeping pill bottle spilled beside her.

"Oh, God! No! Please, Cristy! No!"

Lee knelt beside the motionless form and carefully touched her throat. She had a pulse. Weak. But a pulse. He picked her up and carried her into the living room couch beside the phone. He shook her. Gently at first. Then roughly.

"Cristy! Cristy! Wake up! Talk to me!"

She mumbled something incoherent.

He shouted at her, "Listen to me, honey! You can't sleep now! Wake up and talk to me!"

"...Lee,...I..." She muttered words he could not understand. "...Let me 'lone...want to sleep..."

"No baby! Stay awake! Talk to me while I make a phone call." Trying to shake her with his left hand, he dialed the operator with his right. "Operator! Hospital emergency room . . ."

"Keep her awake. Slap her if you have to, but keep her awake," the emergency room doctor told Lee. "Give her salt and warm water until she throws up. If she doesn't improve, bring her to the emergency room."

Lee held her head when she began to heave. Her body rid itself of the substance she had swallowed. Fortunately her stomach was empty of food since she had not eaten supper. But she wanted to sleep, and the doctor had told Lee to keep her awake for at least eight hours. When her eyelids drooped toward sleep, he shook her—and prodded her with questions to solicit conversation.

"You know I love you, Cristy. You know the kids love you. You do know that, don't you, honey?"

She spoke weakly. He couldn't hear her. "What, Cristy? Don't you know we love you, baby? Talk to me."

". . . children . . . love me . . . Lee. Lee don't love me. Other women . . . lies . . . not true to me."

"Oh, Cristy, please don't say that! There are not other women. I am true to you. I swear! Oh, please, God, let her know how much I love and need her. Please, God, save her. I'll never let anything hurt her again." He pulled her to her feet and began walking her around the room . . . back and forth . . . back and forth . . . until the effects of the pills finally faded and she was totally awake.

Coming out of it, she said, "Oh Lee, how stupid of me. I couldn't get to sleep, and I thought some extra pills might help. I remember getting dizzy and faint after I took them. I couldn't make it back to the bed. I don't know what happened after that." She was totally exhausted. But when Lee's arms went around her, she suddenly tensed and pulled away from him. She did not say anything. She got up silently and went in to check on the children, going from bed to bed to touch the tiny youngsters and adjust their covers. Then she came back into the living room and sat across from Lee. Silent. *I have to think this out,* her mind said to her.

Lee waited.

After a few minutes she said, choosing her words carefully, "Lee, I've been trying for weeks to talk with you about us and about the problems here at home. You just won't listen. I can't take it any more."

He began an apology, but she interrupted him. "Lee, when I married you, I was very, very proud. You were something special. You were my everything. It was like I'd waited for you all my life. Then you let me down when you went to that motel with that other woman."

"Baby, I've told you how sorry I was for that. And I promised you it would never happen again."

She was so intent on what she had to say that she barely heard him. "Then I saw a different person from the one I married." She picked her words precisely. "You were like a stranger to me—and, yet, still the man I married. You left me confused. It was as if my whole life was crumbling before me. I tried to get over it. I believe I really had—and then Roy and Rosalie started poisoning my mind with their talk. Night after night, the same thing. It made me question you all over again."

This time she wanted to hear his answer, and she looked at him intently. Waiting . . .

"Their talk was ridiculous," Lee declared. "I don't know why they would say such things."

"They did, though. They kept telling me in lurid detail about your activity with other girls, Lee. I didn't want to hear it. I told them so. But they wouldn't stop. The same thing, over and over. Lee, I cannot—and will not—live with an unfaithful husband."

"Cristy, I swear to you that I am faithful to you, and that you're the only one I love."

"I want to believe that, Lee."

"You *can* trust me! What can I say or do to prove myself to you?"

"That's going to take time. But I do know one thing. Right now something has to be done about Roy and Rosalie. I can't live like this anymore. When I come home at night I'm exhausted. I don't need the confusion and mess that's here. Nor the accusations against you."

"I'll do something about it!" Lee stated flatly.

"Right away, Lee. I know Roy's your brother, and I don't want to hurt anyone's feelings, but either they go, or I go. It's that simple."

"No choice there. I'll just tell them it's a bit too crowded with two families and six children under one roof."

The next day Lee tried to be diplomatic with Roy. But . . .

"This is Ellie's idea, isn't it, Lee?"

"Cristy, Roy. Cristy's *and my* idea, Roy. Cristy is my wife, and I have to think of her over anyone else."

Roy agreed to move.

11

C risty Lane smiled in the mirror at herself. Approvingly. The face that looked back at her was happy. While she was still not sure she liked herself as a blonde, Lee had insisted she looked great, that being blonde would be good for her singing career. Well, she wasn't sure it looked *that* great, but it was different . . . and kind of fun . . .

A lot had happened during the months since Roy and Rosalie had moved. Lee had changed jobs again —twice. From Watkins he had gone to being a salesman for Montgomery Ward, and then to setting up fund-raising campaigns for various organizations. Which had brought up a more or less standard joking question from Cristy's brothers: "What's Lee doing this week?" As their father had done before them, Cristy's brothers all stayed with one job day-after-day and year-after-year. Lee's moving from job to job puzzled them. Nevertheless, they liked Lee. As for Cristy's singing career, well, that was just plain ridiculous. They couldn't visualize their little sister, the child they had remembered tottering around the kitchen after their mother, being paid to sing. And now this night club thing . . .

Lee had leased the basement of the Jefferson Hotel in Peoria and turned it into their own night club, "Cristy's, Inc. . . ." Cristy sighed. Sometimes it was impossible living with that man! He was just too good at everything he did. He never seemed to fail. *And here I am cringing at the thought of another performance tonight,* she told her image in the mirror. It wasn't just the singing. By now, she really enjoyed singing—although it was never easy performing in front of other people. No . . . *I guess I never feel myself quite capable of doing what Lee expects me to do . . .*

Lee—

An odd thought caught Cristy's mind and pulled her toward the mirror as though it somehow came from her reflected image. *Lee . . . He wants so much from me. What would I do if he left me because I can't make him happy by being what he wants me to be? How would I get along? My life is so intertwined with Lee's . . .*

Yet . . .

That wasn't really the thought . . . not the odd

part. Something was missing. Something was left out . . . some thought she did not want to think . . . could not think . . .

The dull ache throbbing now in her stomach brought her back to reality. "Here we go again," she muttered aloud as she headed toward the bathroom. Her bouts with stomach trouble seemed to be getting worse . . .

"What's the matter, honey?" Lee asked as they drove to the club. "Is it your stomach again?"

"Yes. Same old thing."

"I don't think it's natural, Cristy. And it doesn't seem that any of the doctors you have been to have been able to help. You're always on edge. I think even the kids notice it."

"I'm taking the medicine that's been prescribed for me. And I really have cut down on the colas I've been drinking."

"I think it's more than that, Cristy. A friend of mine told me about the Mayo Clinic. He said they are really thorough there. I think you ought to go."

"Not *another* psychiatrist, Lee. Please! The last one you had me go to did nothing but ask me about my sex life and my mother! Then all she did was give me some more pills."

"The Mayo Clinic is different, baby. You don't just see a psychiatrist, you get a complete physical. Won't you please go for me?"

She was ready to refuse when the pain grabbed

at her stomach, sharper this time. *Maybe* . . . "Okay, I'll go—but on one condition: that you have a checkup, too. You haven't had one in a long time, and the hours you are putting in now would be hard on two men, let alone one."

They both took a week off from work, left the children with the baby-sitter, and headed toward Rochester, Minnesota. The trip turned into a lark. They talked and laughed along the way, and Cristy almost forgot her apprehension about the examination. But once having completed the necessary lab tests and examinations she found her fears returning when she got to the psychiatrist's office.

"How do you feel, Cristy?" Dr. Hawes asked, puffing on a pipe.

"A little nervous."

"More than usual?"

"I guess . . ."

"Are you always nervous and tense?"

"Most of the time." She felt tears unaccountably beginning to sting her eyes, and she swallowed hard to eliminate the lump in her throat.

"It's okay to cry, Cristy. It might be just the thing you need." His voice was gentle, understanding . . .

That did it. All the fears and insecurities she had felt over the years began to well up inside her, and she cried uncontrollably. She reached for a tissue, hoping to stop the tears. It seemed like an eternity before they finally subsided.

"I feel so silly," she said, trying to smile.

The kindly doctor shook his head. "No need for that. Now, why don't you tell me about it?"

"I'm not sure what it is myself. I just feel like I have no control over my life, that no matter what I do it's not good enough. If I say something wrong, Lee gets upset. If I pick out a dress he doesn't like, it goes back to the store. He even tells me what—and how—to eat sometimes!" Cristy paused and reached for another tissue.

"How about the singing, Cristy? Do you like it?"

"At times. Sometimes I do enjoy it. I've always liked to sing. It's just that . . . I'm afraid it's never going to be good enough . . . or that someone will laugh at me when I step on that stage."

"Good enough for whom?"

"Good enough for Lee . . . or the audience, I guess. I just feel so frightened most of the time . . . and unworthy, somehow . . ."

"Mmmm . . ." The doctor nodded his head thoughtfully. "Do you ever tell Lee how you feel?"

"No . . ."

"Do you ever express your opinions on anything to him?"

"Well, . . . sometimes I try . . . But he always seems to have something more important to say. As if he's always right." Then she added quickly, afraid the doctor would get the wrong impression:

"I do love him very much. It's just that he's so sure of himself . . . so positive . . . so outgoing. I'm none of these things. He is so successful in everything he does. He is constantly winning awards for one thing or another. I feel insignificant next to him. I'd never go out and push myself in the way he does. And I certainly would never go after a singing career on my own!"

The doctor got up from his chair and came around to the front of his desk. He knocked his pipe against the ashtray and slowly began to repack it with the tobacco he pulled from his pocket.

"Cristy," he said, looking up at her, "you know, you're a person, too. You have thoughts, ideas, and values just like anyone else. And you certainly must have talent—or the club Lee told me you have would not be doing so well. Those people come to hear you sing. No one forces them to sit and listen to you.

"As for Lee, you have got to start speaking up—unless you want to stay nervous and depressed the rest of your life. You can't possibly please everyone, so you might as well be happy with yourself. If Lee really loves you—and I think he does—he will not leave you because you speak your mind.

"Now, Cristy," he said as he wrote something on a piece of paper, "I am giving you two prescriptions. This first one is to be filled at the drugstore. I want the names of the doctors who gave you those other pills. You should never have been taking that much—not someone as small as you. It's no wonder you were so depressed. Sometimes, when not properly prescribed, these so-called anti-depressants can have the opposite effect."

He tore the sheet from the pad and handed it to Cristy.

"The second prescription is to start reading every self-help book you can get your hands on. Any library or bookstore can provide you with a long list."

His parting command, kindly but firm, as he showed her to the door was, "Remember, there is a very strong and wonderful person inside you. Let her come out, and you'll see you are really never alone."

Before they started back for Peoria, they stopped off at a restaurant, and she noticed that Lee was in particularly good spirits. She watched him pick up a piece of chicken from the plate he had just been served.

"Well," he said expansively, "I got a clean bill of health. Fit as a fiddle. What did the doctor have to say to you, my dear?"

Cristy took a sip of her hot tea. *Now, Lee, how are you going to take what I have to tell you?* She reached for a chicken leg on her plate and started to answer him. "Well, I have to get new medicine. And he advised me to get some self-help books. And, Lee—"

"Honey, don't eat that chicken with your fingers. It just doesn't look right."

That did it.

Suddenly she was no longer afraid of how Lee would handle what she couldn't hold back. But she did try to keep her voice under control. "That's the main thing the doctor said! You have got to quit telling me what to say! What to do! How to act! How to eat! You are eating your own chicken with your fingers, and if you say one more word about how I should eat mine, I will get up and walk out of here right now."

Once started, she felt as though she couldn't stop. She felt set free . . .

"You have got to let me speak my mind, Lee. I am a person too—but sometimes I think you forget that. You like to control things. Well, I'm not a thing, and you cannot control me. I can't let you any longer."

She looked at Lee imploringly and reached across the table to touch his hand. "Lee, I do love you. But things have got to change. I cannot be afraid that you are going to leave me every time we have an argument, or any time I want to speak my mind."

How was he taking it? She saw him staring back at her across the table . . .

On the trip back to Peoria Cristy felt a lifting sense of relief. The very world itself seemed

brighter than it had in years. *I am my own person
. . .* Well, maybe a little shaky . . . but confident that
she could stand on her own two feet no matter
what. It was a great feeling.

The movement of the car down the highway
lulled her, and bits of daydreams floated in her consciousness. One stayed—the memory of the Sunday
when she was 17 and had gone to church with Carol
Hatcher, her best friend . . . After all these years
Cristy could not remember the details, the why or
how, but she could remember the feeling . . . the
quiet strength as she listened to the sermon. God
had been with her then . . .

God . . .

The psychiatrist hadn't said anything about religion.

*Maybe because that's something I have to take care of
all by myself . . . and in my own way . . .*

Still . . .

The memory of the warm feeling of having God
with her came flooding back over the years.

Cristy smiled as she looked out the car window.
God is with me now . . .

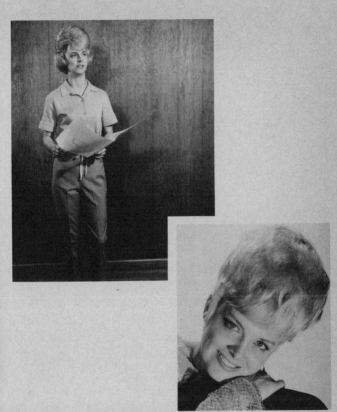

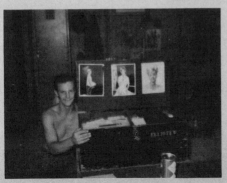

Cristy's brother Charlie.

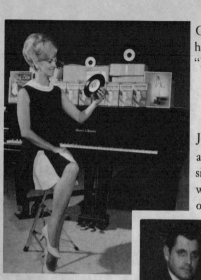

Cristy looks at
her first record,
"I'm Saving My Kisses."

John Talley, Cristy,
and John Elgin, V.P.,
signing a record contract
with Spar before leaving
on tour to Vietnam.

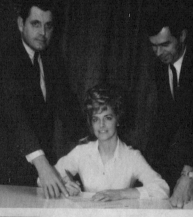

Cristy, Cindy,
Tammy, Kevin.

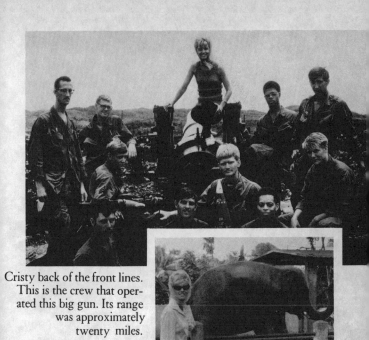

Cristy back of the front lines. This is the crew that operated this big gun. Its range was approximately twenty miles.

Cristy at the Saigon Zoo.

Cristy and GIs at Da Nang.

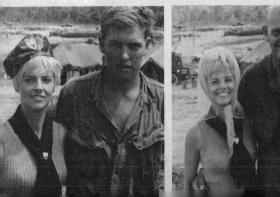

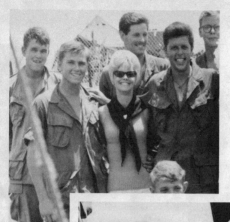

Cristy always
took time for
pictures
with GIs.

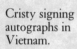

Cristy signing
autographs in
Vietnam.

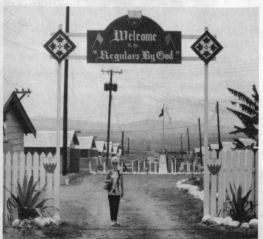

Cristy Lane.

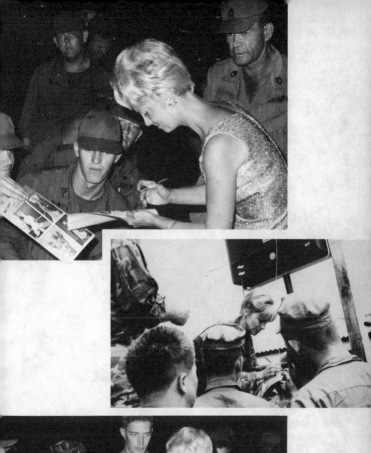
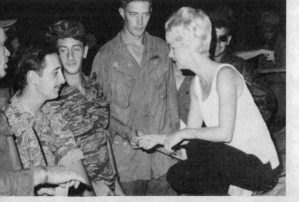

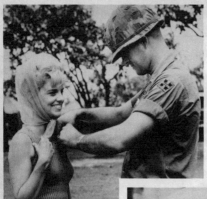

Cristy received
a medal.

Cristy in
Saigon taxi.

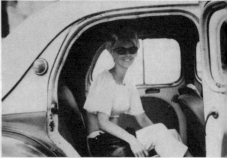

Cristy in Vietnam.

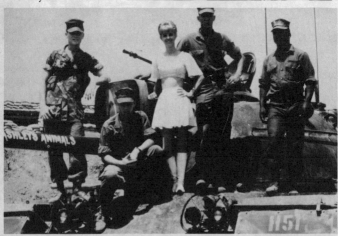

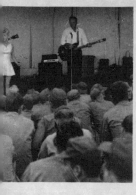

Cristy.

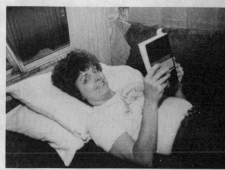

Cristy relaxing
on the bus.

Cristy leaving
the hospital in Saigon.

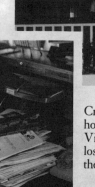

Cristy after returning
home from 120 shows in
Vietnam where she almost
lost her life, looks over
the mail.

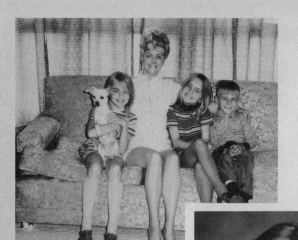

Cindy, Kurly, Cristy,
Tammy, and Kevin.

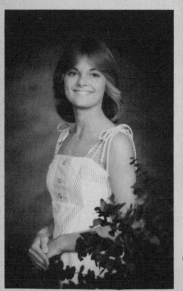

Tammy's graduation picture —
1978, Madison High School.

Cynthia's graduation picture—
1979, Madison High School.

12

The year was 1969, and Cristy knew that it was going to be a good one. At least she *thought* it was going to be a good one this particular evening as she busied herself in the kitchen waiting for Lee to return from a business trip.

She really enjoyed singing now. And she had put into practice much of what she had learned at the Mayo Clinic. No longer was she letting Lee make *all* the decisions. She had put her foot down a time or two when his schemes had been just a little bit too hare-brained. She was learning to form her own decisions, make up her own mind. Well, . . . most of the time. Oddly, being independent had seemed to give her even greater respect for Lee's abilities. Besides, she loved him.

But the singing. That now was a joy instead of a fearful ordeal. She supposed having her own band, "The Misty Men," helped—even if her front man, Billy Arr, had left for Topeka, Kansas where he had purchased his own night club. She had even taken in stride the change in her own club. The Jefferson Hotel had been turned into a nursing home, thus ending Lee's lease for "Cristy's, Inc."—but they now had a new club,

"The Flame," where Cristy performed . . . whenever she wasn't booked at a fair or military base. Actually, it was all . . . kinda fun . . .

She heard a car in the driveway and looked out the window to see Lee's big Lincoln Continental. *We are doing well,* she thought.

Lee was smiling as he walked into the kitchen. He seemed, well, just a little happier than usual— and that should have tipped her off that he was up to something. But—

"Hello, honey." He kissed her and slipped his arms around her waist. "How's my girl?"

"Just fine. How was your trip?"

"Great. Just great."

It was the little pause that came next that made her smell a mouse. *Lee Stoller, what are you planning for me now?*

"Cristy, how would you like to go to Vietnam?" *Did I hear him right?* "Vietnam?"

"Yeah. The sergeant I spoke to in Huntsville said we could make some real money by playing service clubs over there. Besides, we'd be doing something for the boys. Good entertainment is scarce there."

"You're *not* kidding, are you?"

"Why, no, my dear. I think it would be great exposure for you. Look at all the publicity Bob Hope gets."

"You really mean it, don't you?"

"Sure."

"You think I could just pack a bag and leave? Lee,

we have children, remember? Tammy. Cindy. Kevin. In case you've forgotten."

"Yeah. We also have a live-in housekeeper and baby-sitter. Ethel's good with the kids. You told me so yourself. She already keeps them while you're at work. And on weekends when we have a gig. What's the difference? Wouldn't be all that long."

"How long?"

"Only about three months."

"Three months!"

"Yeah."

"Three months . . . Lee, I don't know if I would feel right leaving the kids that long. And, Vietnam —isn't it dangerous?"

"Oh, the kids will be fine. And we'll call them often. And if I thought there was any danger to you, I would never even consider it."

"Well . . . You know I trust your judgment. If you think it important that I go, I'll go . . ."

In February, 1969 Lee flew to Vietnam to make the necessary arrangements for her tour. She understood from Lee that she would be booked in various service clubs around Vietnam, with Saigon as the home base. Payment would depend upon the decision of a government panel which would decide how much they were worth after hearing the whole band, but Lee assured her they would get top dollar.

When Lee returned, they got ready in a hectic

two weeks. Lee bought round-trip tickets for Cristy, the band, and himself. They rushed their passports. They got their shots. Everything was set.

Except—

At the last minute the band changed their minds. Only a week before the plane was to take off.

That, thought Cristy, *is the end of that.* But Lee got on the phone to Nashville, found an agent with a band eager and ready to go. There wouldn't be time for rehearsal, but if the band was sent some tapes of Cristy's material they would have it learned by the time they all got to Vietnam. "Don't worry," the agent told Lee. "The band is great."

For Cristy, leaving wasn't all that great . . . the lump in her throat . . . waving to the three unhappy faces as the car pulled away from the curb . . . the lurch of the huge 707 into the air . . . Nashville to St. Louis . . . to San Francisco . . . to Hawaii . . . to Guam . . . to the Philippines. Soon they would be in Saigon.

"Would you care for something to eat, ma'am?" the flight attendant asked.

"No thank you . . ." Not on a nervous stomach, no matter how hungry she was. She wished she could be as calm as Lee. There he was, just calmly shuffling papers in his briefcase . . . *as if he were going to another business meeting . . .* She opened her book and tried to read. Eventually she dozed off. A voice on the intercom woke her.

". . . your captain. We are approaching Saigon airport and should touch down in five minutes. Please fasten your seat belts and put up the folding table in front of you. Secure any loose objects, and, when the light comes on and you hear the buzzer, lean forward and put your head between your knees."

Cristy looked over at Lee . . . puzzled . . .

"Due to increased hostilities," the captain continued, "the airfield has a fire zone, and this plane will free fall several miles to pass quickly through the danger of being hit by enemy fire. You may experience an uncomfortable feeling for a brief time, but we do expect a safe landing."

Now she really was frightened. "Lee, you didn't tell me it was like this."

"It wasn't when I flew over." He reached for her hand.

The buzzer sounded. The flashing light came on. The plane turned on its side. The engine seemed to stall. The huge aircraft dropped like a dead weight through the sky. The earth rushed toward them at what seemed to Cristy alarming speed. They fell until she was sure they would crash. Then the jet engines roared back to life, and the plane began to glide safely toward earth.

Cristy breathed a sigh of relief. *Am I glad I turned down that food!* she thought. She turned toward Lee. Even his face looked a little green, and what was apparently intended to be a reassuring smile for her turned out to be a sort of half-hearted sick grin. She had to laugh. "Didn't a certain man tell me this flight would be as comfortable as sitting on our living room sofa?"

"Right this minute that's exactly where I wish we were."

Saigon airport was small compared to the other airfields they had seen during their trip. Cristy noticed military vehicles and troops moving out about the buildings. *You sure can tell the difference between the American buildings and the Vietnamese ones*, she thought as she looked out her window before deplaning. The American structures were fairly new and well-kept in comparison to the run-down, neglected Vietnamese buildings.

Cristy caught her breath as she stepped outside. The 110-degree heat was stifling. The humidity was so thick it was hard to breathe. She looked around her—and suddenly her heart skipped a beat.

Standing there was Charlie, her brother.

"Hi, Sis," Charlie said as he hugged her tightly. "I just got me a 10-day furlough, so I thought I'd show you the sights before your tour starts."

Cristy was glad to have Charlie along as they bounced down the streets of Saigon in the van that Ladd Productions, the agency handling their tour, had provided. Charlie was a steady influence, helping her stand the shock of what she saw. Saigon. It looked more like Skid Row. Worse, maybe, for even the poorest sections of Peoria looked warm and cozy by comparison to the huts these people called home. It was the children that got to Cristy most . . . small children with sparrow-like arms and legs . . . stomachs swollen from hunger . . . weather-ragged skirts . . . big, solemn eyes watching the van pass . . . But the adults were pitiful, too. Scrawny men with hardly a stitch of clothing were sleeping in the dirt roads. Then Cristy gasped as she saw a man idly relieve himself in the street.

"That's normal, Cristy," her brother said in response to her horrified expression. "And do you notice there aren't many dogs running around loose? Too valuable. They're the main course over here. That's how poor this country is."

At the Ladd office, Cristy was thankful she had brought her overnight case with her on the plane. Neither their luggage nor their band equipment had arrived—probably wouldn't for several days. She was tired now. And hungry. She wanted to get something to eat and get to the hotel so she could try to relax. The agency offered them the rooms they normally provided free of charge for all their acts, but Lee declined, having seen what they were like on his previous trip. He booked rooms for them at the Park Hotel, the second-best in the country. It was just two blocks from the Presidential palace.

On the way to the hotel they stopped to get something to eat. Cristy only picked at the lukewarm wieners and beans, the best that the so-called restaurant had to offer. If this was any indication of the food she was going to be living on, she didn't know what she was going to do.

The desk clerk at the hotel gave Lee's party three rooms and charged him $500 a week. The clerk pointed the way to the stairs, saying that sometimes the self-service elevator didn't work.

"Well, here's home for the next three months," Lee said, opening the door to their hotel room.

Cristy stood at the threshold, staring in disbelief.

The room was smaller than any she had ever stayed in. It was also hotter. The air conditioner that buzzed noisily in the corner did nothing but stir up the already stale and humid air. A single light bulb hung from its socket in the ceiling, a pull chain dangling beneath it. A chipped porcelain lamp stood by the narrow bed. The bathroom had cracked and protruding tile.

Cristy turned to Lee, her nose wrinkled in distaste. "If this is the second-best in Saigon, I'd hate to see the worst."

"I'm sorry, baby. But it is war country."

He looked so forlorn she reached over to give him a kiss.

But she didn't make it—

A loud series of *cracks!* came from outside.

Cristy jumped.

"What's that?"

"Just a little shooting. Probably on the outskirts

of town. I understand the Vietcong try to sneak in around sundown."

"Are we safe?"

"Of course we are, honey."

Relieved, she went to the window. She noticed streaks of light crossing the sky, leaving a trail of fire. Rockets. As they hit the ground she saw them explode only blocks away. Stifling a cry, she pointed outside to Lee.

"It wasn't like this a few weeks ago," Lee said, startled. He called the desk clerk.

"The Vietcong," the clerk explained, "slip in close to the city at night and fire rockets at the Presidential palace, then steal back to the jungle at dawn to keep from being sighted. But, don't worry. No rockets have landed near the hotel in over a week."

Over a week? Cristy lay wide-eyed in Lee's arms while the explosions went on, long into the night. It was hours before, exhausted, she finally fell into a restless sleep . . .

The Cristy Lane Show's first schedule was a 17-day tour of Long Bien, a 20-mile drive from Saigon. Each morning they were to load up the Ladd van and travel to each show . . . strategically sandwiched in between military jeeps and armed trucks for protection. Each evening they would return to Saigon the same way.

Cristy was nervous as she heard Lee begin his introduction for her first Vietnam show. It wasn't the thousand or more GI's in front of the stage bothering her right now. It was the band. Neither she nor Lee had believed their ears when they held their first rehearsal a few days ago. Nobody in the band seemed to be playing the same song. Before, Russell, the bandleader and rhythm guitar player, had kept telling Lee how the band had Cristy's material down pat from the tapes Lee had sent them. He bragged that none of them could read music, that they played by ear.

Apparently not the same ear, though. Flo, Russell's wife and the drummer for the group, pounded out one beat on her drums while Russell whanged out another rhythm on his guitar. Only Mike, the bass player, and Paul, the lead guitarist, were even nearly passable.

Lee was so upset he told Cristy he would cancel the whole tour were it not for the fact that now they couldn't afford not to go on. Instead, he just told the band to play very, very softly and let Cristy's voice dominate the sound. It worked. The next day the panel of government officials who reviewed the acts for the service clubs and set the price gave them top-dollar—$500 for large clubs and $300 for small clubs. So here they were . . .

Cristy said a quick prayer to herself as she heard Lee finish his introduction: "I've introduced many entertainers in my time, but not one has given me the honor and pleasure it does to introduce to you this lovely young lady. She sings them all. She sings them her way, and apparently that is the right way. Please make welcome . . . the lovely and talented . . . Cristy Lane!"

The applause was deafening as Cristy walked onto the stage. Her nervousness began to subside as she looked out at the weary faces of the soldiers. She had never seen an audience so attentive . . .

She sang songs about love . . . and heartbreak . . . and home. So, for a little while they could all forget about the war and their surroundings.

When she finished, she got the first of what would add up to over 300 standing ovations. She was brought back for five encores before she finally stopped and stepped down to sign autographs. It was only then that she realized what effect her being there had on the men. They milled around her, talking and laughing and shaking her hand. Some just wanted to be near someone from home. Others wanted to touch her. And some had not been around a woman with round eyes in so long that they were almost afraid of her.

"Ma'am, would you mind if I had my picture taken with you?" one young GI asked timidly. "I sure would love to send it to the folks back home."

"Why, surely." Cristy smiled into the boy's face. *He doesn't look old enough to shave,* she thought to herself as she put her arm around his waist to pose for the picture. Immediately, she felt his body tense, and she realized he was afraid to touch her. She smiled reassuringly. "It's okay, soldier. I won't bite."

The young man gingerly slipped his arm around her, and another soldier took the picture. Cristy tried not to notice how uncontrollably the boy's hand shook as it touched her. *Poor kid* . . .

Another soldier came up to her and said bashfully, "I haven't seen an American girl in so long I've forgotten what one looks like." He turned to Lee. "Could I have your permission to kiss her—on the cheek, that is?"

Lee laughed warmly. "Sure, soldier, go ahead."

When the crowd finally thinned out, Cristy realized she was starving. She had always made it a practice never to eat before a performance, with the result that she was very hungry afterwards. Now, since they were not with the USO, they had to find their own meals, and they ended up at a tent that served as a makeshift kitchen.

Cristy looked down at the food she was served: hot dogs, beans, and the inevitable rice. Not very appetizing, but she was so hungry she thought even this would taste good. But— After she had eaten a few bites of her rice she noticed tiny little black specks on her plate. The specks moved. Cristy stared at them. In wide-eyed horror . . .

Ants!

The rice had ants in it!

She pushed her plate of food away.

She was no longer hungry. But she did have one satisfaction: the soldiers had been the best audience she had ever had . . .

The days that followed began to run into one another. Cristy and her group packed and unpacked equipment in what seemed an endless cycle of different locations. Sometimes they did as many as five shows in one day, traveling in convoys through the jungle. Always there was the blistering heat and the fine hot sand that blew incessantly. Always there was the bad water and the poor food. It all began to show on Cristy. Ever since the ants-in-the-food episode at Long Bien she had not been able to eat much. She was losing weight fast. Her clothes were beginning to look as though they were simply hanging on her. Only another woman would understand the feeling *that* gave her . . .

At Bien Hoa where she was to perform that afternoon, she eyed the show site with the now-familiar feeling of dismay. *Another outside performance under the hot sun* . . . A huge wooden stage had been erected in an open field on the very edge of the jungle. Several thousand troops sat on row-after-row of wooden benches. Not a blade of grass stirred in the dense heat.

Yet, as Cristy walked out on the stage, all the unpleasantness vanished. She enjoyed singing to these men. During the past several weeks she had begun to feel a quiet bond developing between them and her as she sang. She forgot the heat . . . and her tired body . . .

Suddenly there was a thundering roar.

Cristy looked up to see an Air Force jet firing its guns into the grass near the jungle, not 500 feet away. Other jets followed, shooting into the grass and dropping small bombs.

Cristy glanced at Lee, and at the men sitting out front. Not one of the men even flinched. The only movement any of them made was toward her, to hear her song better.

She kept on singing.

When she finished, the applause was deafening, and the GI's leaped to their feet in tribute to her courage.

She finished the performance as though nothing had happened.

13

S ometimes, though . . .
    Like that return to Long Bien, and
    evening performance, scheduled out-
doors . . .

Again, over a thousand soldiers packed the benches. Floodlights bathed the stage, and it seemed to Cristy she could feel the heat of them washing over her blonde hair, her silver mini-skirt, her boots. The band's instruments glittered, sending off sparks of light that moved in time with the music.

Cristy finished her last number and stood on the outside of the stage talking with Arnold, a young private who had been assigned as her escort, while Russell sang a novelty song as part of the show. Lee was on the other side of the stage, separated from her.

Suddenly a siren wailed.

"The camp is under attack, Miss Cristy," Arnold told her. "Come with me. Quickly, please. The camp will be blacked out. I have to get you to cover."

She caught only a faint glimpse of Lee in the moving crowd as the lights faded and died. Faint moonlight covered the soldiers. Cristy was amazed that everyone seemed to know just where to go in the near-total darkness. Her heart beat faster as she heard guns firing. There seemed to be explosions all over the camp. *I wish I had Lee* . . . But she let Arnold lead her into the darkness of a large barracks where there were others. She realized she was totally separated not only from Lee but also from the band. She was holding tightly to Arnold's hand. She couldn't control her trembling.

The unseen soldiers around them laughed and cracked jokes. *Are they used to this? Or is it just their way of relieving the tension?* She felt oddly uncomfortable. As though in danger . . .

"You know, it's been ten months since I've seen a woman," Arnold said, squeezing Cristy's hand. She sensed an undertone in his voice. "You just put yourself in my hands, and I'll take care of you."

She knew what he meant . . . But she didn't want to believe it.

Then he put his arm around her small shoulders and pulled her a little closer to him.

Lee! she thought frantically—as though the thought would bring him here to protect her. *Oh, Lee!* She felt small and helpless. She did not know what to do. What if the attack lasted all night? What if Arnold . . .

It seemed like an eternity before the lights finally came back on. Yet it was not until Lee walked in the door that Arnold dropped his arm from around her.

Cristy breathed a sigh of relief. "Oh Lee! I was

beginning to think I might not see you again." Eagerly, she took his arm. *I love you, Lee Stoller . . . even if you do get me in the worst predicaments . . .*

"Honey, I had no idea things would be this bad when I contracted this tour. Just say the word, and we'll go home."

"No. We made a commitment." She did not tell him about Arnold. But Lee had an odd look on his face. *I wonder what he's thinking . . .*

She could not read his mind. What he was really thinking at that moment concerned what he had heard about another entertainer, Jeanie Black, who had been shot through the head by a sniper while singing for an audience. Lee was not one given to praying. But . . .

Several days later the caravan headed back to Saigon. They finished their shows at Bien Hoa by midafternoon and joined the early convoy back to Long Bien. From there they were to merge with a large group going into Saigon. The caravan moved steadily along. There had been no trouble, and they were relatively relaxed. Ahead was a slight rise in the roadway. Tall jungle grass stretched out on each side to meet the forest.

The young GI who manned the machine gun on the jeep in front of the Ladd van had been to several of Cristy's shows, and his was now a familiar face. A friendly, likable face. He had a cowlick. The makings of a natural comedian. He had pushed his steel helmet at a rakish angle to one side, and he was clowning around for the band's benefit, making faces and swinging his arms wide, pretending he was singing for an audience. One hand was still on the machine gun mounted on the rear of the Jeep, but his eyes were on the band—his audience.

Cristy laughed. "A man with that much talent, Lee, we should put him on our next show."

The sound of her voice had not died in her mind when the smile on the boy's face froze.

Bullets were ripping through his body, their impact jerking him back. He slumped over the gun he had been strapped to. He was dead.

It happened so suddenly, it was such a shock to her mind, that Cristy could not believe it. She sat motionless. Surely she would wake from the nightmare.

But blood was staining the dead boy's uniform, and, three vehicles ahead of her own van, another van burst into flames from a direct rocket hit.

She felt Lee's hands grab her and push her to the van floor. Yet she could still see a slice of the sky upward through the van's window and the section of forest from which the attack had come. The Vietcong fire was spraying the convoy, and rockets sent smoke and debris everywhere. But within moments the weapons from the convoy centered on the area in the jungle from which the attack had come, the section of forest she could see, and there was an enormous thundering of firepower . . . and the forest in her vision ceased to exist—trees, grass, everything bursting skyward.

The attack from the unseen enemy was silenced, and the skirmish ended as abruptly as it had started.

But the young boy was dead.

It was the first time she had seen violent death . . . a life forever ended . . .

It was dark when they neared Saigon. The Ladd driver, still shaken from the day's events, missed his turn toward the Park Hotel. A South Vietnamese army truck blocked the way as he tried to turn around. Soldiers piled out of the truck and surrounded the Ladd van; guns waving menacingly. None of them spoke English, and the Ladd driver could not explain who they were nor where they were headed.

Flo began to scream.

Cristy was silent. The nightmare of the day had drained her of all response.

A half hour later an English-speaking officer finally arrived to clear them.

Not until she was back at the hotel and had curled up next to Lee in bed did Cristy let go. Only then did she begin to cry.

Softly . . . in the darkness . . .

The following morning they were scheduled for a show in the Long Bien area, but when Lee called for the Ladd van, the clerk told him it would not be coming. The Vietcong had overrun Long Bien the day before. Fierce fighting was still going on. It was a blood bath. Hundreds of Americans were killed.

The news stunned Cristy and Lee. They had made many friends among the GI's there. Now . . . how many were dead?

There was a lesser problem. "The shows have been cancelled for a week, Cristy," Lee said. She saw the worried look on his face and realized it was better for her own peace of mind to worry about this rather than about the deaths . . . She knew the figures as well as Lee—a week's cancellation would cost them personally at least $5,000 . . .

"Well," Lee said, "we may as well take a tour of Saigon today."

It seemed to Cristy that the dirty city was even dirtier than on the day they had arrived, and the people even poorer. The cab drove them up and down the streets, and she watched in horror as she saw children and adults alike rummaging inside a garbage truck for food. At that moment an emaciated Vietnamese woman came to the window of the cab. She held a small baby wrapped in torn blankets.

"Give a good home in 'Merica," she pleaded in broken English as she held the baby in outstretched arms toward Cristy. "We starve here. Please, kind lady."

It was too much for Cristy.

She swallowed hard and looked at Lee. He ordered the taxi to drive them back to their hotel. The two of them spent the rest of the week at the hotel.

To keep the band in practice—and, Cristy guessed, to keep her own mind off the lizards crawling freely about the restaurant walls and the ants marching across the tables in search of sugar bowls —Lee scheduled several free shows at the hotel's Rooftop Club, patronized by wealthier Vietnamese and some American officers.

Lee became friends with one regular patron, an American colonel who arrived early and drank late —and who had definite opinions about the Vietnam War.

"It's a crime, Lee, of international proportions. None of us really understand why we are here. I've been in the military nearly 30 years—through World War II, in Korea, now here in 'Nam. We can't win this war. When the enemy attacks, often we can't even fire back without calling headquarters and getting permission. They like to attack us and hide in the rice paddies. If we mess up the rice paddies, the American government has to pay for the damaged crops. I can't condemn the Americans who rebel against this war. It's a situation created to line the pockets of a few. Large corporations are becoming multimillionaires over it. Our boys are being killed, maimed, and forgotten in the jungles here."

They talked often. Lee heard the same comments from other Americans, both military and civilian.

"Saigon is a filthy place," one American said. "Life expectancy here is 34 years. But compared to the rest of the country, Saigon is Broadway."

"I've noticed that," Lee replied. "We have a lot of shows left to do out in the boondocks when the cancellation ends."

"The rest of the shows are still going on. They have some big-name stars here in Saigon tonight."

"That's the difference," Lee replied. "The government runs the USO. They take good care of them. Keep them a long way from the fighting."

"You're not with the USO?"

"No. We're with the service clubs. They're self-supporting. And they're located everywhere. Anywhere there's a GI."

After six days and an estimated loss of $5,000, Cristy went back to work, picking up the schedule from the next show date. An Army C-47 took the troupe the short 150-mile trip from Saigon to Da Nang. From the plane, Cristy could see a muddy river weaving through the conglomeration of small and large wooden and masonry buildings which was home to 200,000 people. A few scattered trees thrust green fists up from the dust of the dirt streets. There were only two paved streets in the entire city.

The heat is even worse here, Cristy thought as she

climbed down from the C-47. Her clothes were clinging to her, and she was anxious to get to the hotel where reservations had already been made for them by Ladd Productions. But, once there, she could not believe her eyes. The room looked like it had never been cleaned. A thick film of grime covered everything from the bed to the ceiling. Roaches crawled up the walls. Mice scampered freely across the floor. It was not livable, but the desk clerk would not refund their money. Lee finally arranged accommodations at the International House and Hospital. Here the ground floor was a hospital, and the second was reserved for wealthy Vietnamese. Cristy and her party had three rooms—and a kitchen where they could cook their own meals.

She lay in bed that night staring up at the ceiling, her nightgown clinging to her because of the humidity. There was no air conditioning. A lonely fan hung from the ceiling, barely stirring the stale air. Louvered slats were the only source of ventilation, but they were an open invitation for insects and lizards.

She turned her head as Lee came into the room. "Where have you been?"

"Oh, just taking a tour of our kitchen. I hope you can get used to buffalo meat—because that's the only change we're going to have from hot dogs. I hear it's kinda tough. But maybe it won't be too bad."

"Was there anything else out there?"

"Some rotten eggs. But I threw them out." He decided not to tell her about the rats he had seen. They were as big as cats and acted like they owned the place, climbing over the table and shelves. But, as he undressed, he did tell her something else. "You know, I had the strangest feeling out there. Like I was being watched."

"Did you see anybody?"

"No. It was too dark. Probably just my imagination." He crawled into bed. "Let's go to sleep."

Cristy rolled over and pulled the thin sheet up to her waist. Suddenly she felt something on her leg. She screamed and kicked.

"What in the world?" Lee jumped out of bed and turned on the light. He looked at the place on the bed where Cristy had been lying. She saw it, too. A lizard. "There's your culprit." Lee laughed. "And, look. You kicked off its tail."

She didn't find that funny. "Well, do something with it. Please, Lee." While he was taking it outside she shook out the bed sheets.

Last time I get into bed without checking it first . . .

The following morning, as the band loaded up the equipment for the day's show, Lee again had the strange feeling he was being watched. It was starting to get on his nerves, and he decided that when they came back that night he was going to do something about it. He did. When they returned after

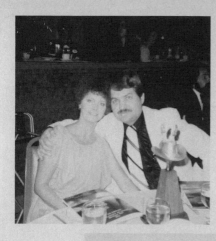

Cristy and Lee after
Cristy won Top
New Female Artist.

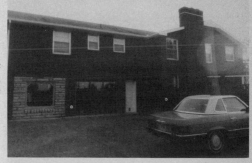

Cristy's garage
has just been
converted to her
private office.

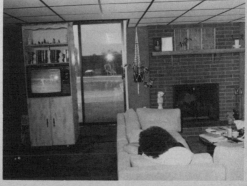

Cristy relaxing
at home, Madison,
Tennessee.

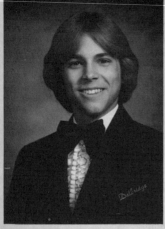

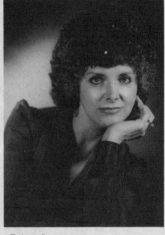

Kevin's graduation picture—
1981, Madison High School.

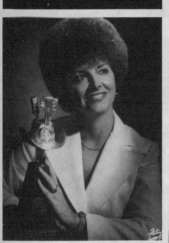

Cristy Lane—
Top New Female Artist—
1979, ACM.

Cristy and Lee's office,
Madison, Tennessee.

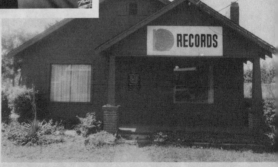

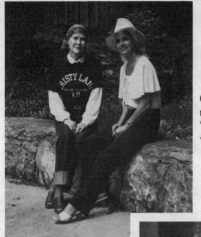

Cristy and Marijohn Wilkin,
the writer of
"One Day at a Time"
with Kristofferson.

Rob Walker, Lee, Cristy,
Don Grierson, V.P. of
United Artists, Cristy's
first gold record
award from New Zealand
for "One Day at a Time."

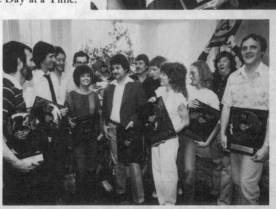

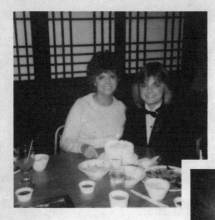

Cristy celebrating
her birthday with Cindy,
January 8, 1983.

Kevin and Mary.

Kevin and Mary's wedding
picture, April 26, 1982.
Lee, Cristy, Mary,
Kevin, Cindy, Tammy.

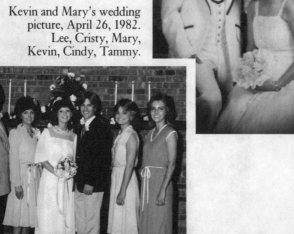

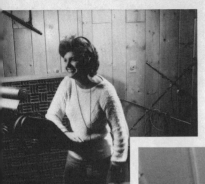

Cristy recording
Christmas album, 1983.

Cristy and
Don Drysdale.
A game between the
California Angels
and Boston Red Sox,
play by play, 1979.

Karen, Cristy, Stacey.
Cristy's first show after
Lee's return,
February 26–27,
1983, the St. Louis
Variety Club Telethon.

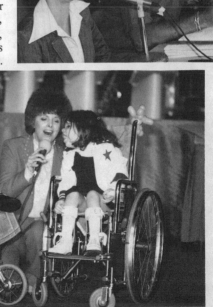

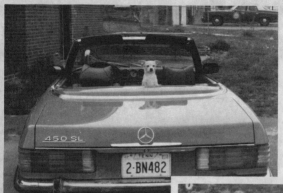

Cristy's 450 SL Mercedes
with Kurly.

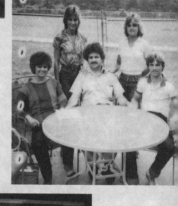

Cristy, Tammy, Lee, Cindy,
Kevin, Maxwell Prison, 1982.

Lee's dad, Lester, eighty years old,
March 13, 1983. Lee,
Cristy, Les, Rory.

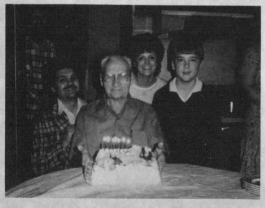

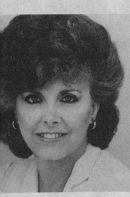

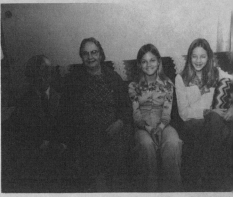

Our favorite Aunt Edna,
the finest Christian we know.

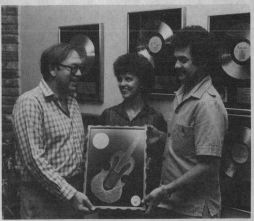

Number one Gospel Album in the World—Cristy
receiving a special award for her *One Day at a Time*
album. Sold over one million and still selling at a
rapid pace worldwide. Lynn Shults, VP Liberty
Records, Cristy, Lee. On the wall displayed are six
more gold and platinum album awards from around
the world for *One Day at a Time*.

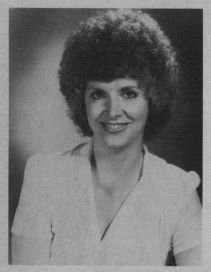

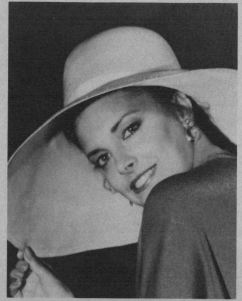

the show, Lee, armed with a flashlight, waited patiently on the kitchen balcony.

Finally he heard a slight stirring behind him. His heart racing, he pulled around and aimed the flashlight at the noise. But all he could see was a small, blurred figure running away in the darkness.

Cristy was with Lee the next day when they did come face to face with the mysterious figure.

"Well," Lee laughed, "there's my ghost." He pointed to a little Vietnamese boy standing at the end of the hallway. Cristy's heart went out to the child, and she smiled reassuringly at him. He had huge, sad brown eyes, and his skinny arms and legs protruded from the rag that was supposed to be his clothing. Before she had a chance to say a word he was off and running.

"Find out about him, Lee," she begged.

Lee asked around. The boy was about six. He had lost both parents in the war, and one of the families staying at the hotel had given him a corner of their room to sleep in. His meals were leftovers from whatever anyone could spare. His bed was a blanket someone had given him. His name was Kam.

The next time Lee saw the kid he tried to offer him a candy bar, but Kam simply ran away. Lee left the candy bar at Kam's door. When that disappeared, he left others. Eventually Kam became more and more responsive. He even ate with Cristy and Lee on occasion in the kitchen, and he delighted in the colorful pictures in the American comic books that Cristy gave him. But he couldn't speak English, so the only way they could communicate was through facial expression and sign language.

His presence got to Cristy.

The day they were to perform at the Acey Deucy Club, Kam, as usual, waved goodbye as the Ladd van pulled away from the hotel. Cristy smiled and waved back, knowing that he would be there to greet them when they returned . . . no matter how late.

"He is so cute," she said to Lee. "I wish there was something we could do for him." Holding Kam in her lap that morning had made her miss her own children even more. She remembered their last phone call to the States and how the children kept asking her when she was coming home.

Homesick for her own children, Cristy glanced idly out the window of the van as the caravan came to a halt. She knew they were to join another convoy to cross the city because the Vietcong guerrillas had infiltrated Da Nang and every precaution had to be taken to protect them against a possible attack.

Ahead, at the bridge, a tall, athletic sentry was checking every vehicle, then waving it across the bridge. *He's the perfect picture of the American GI,* Cristy thought. She was sitting on the front seat of the van with Lee, and she felt pride in the American Army as they watched the procedure. The sentry waved the truck in front of them on, and then turned to their van. Cristy could see his pleasant face.

She heard the rifle shot, cracking above the drone of the motor.

She saw the hole appear in the helmet of the sentry.

His body twisted from the impact and dropped to the ground.

"Stop!" Cristy yelled at their driver. "We've got to help him!" But the van rolled on.

"We can't," the driver explained. "That's up to the military. Our orders are to keep going, no matter what happens. They'll do what they can to help him."

"Oh, Lee!" She grabbed his hands, sinking her own nails deep into his flesh, but not aware of it. "Somebody ought to stop and do what they can . . ."

Lee was trying to soothe her.

He could not . . .

The Acey Deucy Club was a huge building, crowded, and Cristy looked out at the faces before her, gloom darkening her heart. *I wonder how many of you will be alive next week . . . or even tonight . . .* she thought. It was all so senseless . . . a world where sudden violence erased life . . . without warning, apology, or logic. She had never known such a world existed. War. It was not the same as reading about it in the history books . . .

or reading the casualty statistics in the newspaper.
    She sang.
    Applause met the close of each number. When
she asked for requests, one young soldier yelled:
" 'God Bless America,' Cristy! 'God Bless America'." Others chimed in with the same.
    Cristy turned to the band. "Well, guys, think we
can do that one?"
    Paul spoke up. "I've heard it often enough, but
I've never really played it. But I'll give it a try."
    Cristy turned back to the audience. "Fellas, we've
never done this one before. But we'll do the best we
can."
    "That's good enough for us!" a soldier yelled.
    His voice was young . . . vibrant . . . Images
crowded Cristy's brain: the cowlicked machinegunner . . . the young sentry . . .
    "I'd like to dedicate this song . . . to a young
sentry we saw killed on our way here today . . . to
all Americans who have given their lives for their
country . . . to each and every one of you . . ."
    With Paul's guitar as her only accompaniment
she started to sing . . . But the images would not
leave her mind . . .
    Pain and suffering . . . the sentry again . . . again
the young GI who had made her laugh on the ride
back from Long Bien . . . the gaunt faces she had
passed in the streets of Saigon . . . the longing and
loneliness in the eyes of orphaned little boys like
Kam . . . and a room full of tired soldiers fighting

for a war many of them did not understand . . .

Her voice began to waver.

She tried very hard not to cry.

But the images would not go away. And the tears came. She broke. She walked over to the side of the stage to compose herself. Lee handed her a handkerchief.

"You okay, baby?"

She nodded and returned to the center of the stage, but she could only sing a few more lines before she faltered again. Paul continued to strum his guitar, hoping she would recover.

She was sobbing quietly now, unable to sing at all.

The young GI who had made the request came to his feet and began singing himself, his tenor voice at first soft, then growing in intensity: ". . . and stand beside her . . ."

Another voice joined in: ". . . and guide her . . ."

The band members were crying openly now, too.

And Lee . . . Through her own tears Cristy saw that Lee, her own tough Lee, had misty eyes . . .

When she walked off stage, there was thunderous applause.

I am not alone . . . she thought.

Later, when she was composed, Lee told her what one of the sergeants had said to him:

"Lee, I'm not a country music fan, but, I tell you

the truth, that's the finest singer I have ever seen. I've been in the military 25 years, and I've never seen any entertainer get an ovation like this! And . . . she deserves every second of it."

14

T rouble. It seemed to Cristy that after every mountaintop experience there was a deep valley. Again the shows were cancelled for a week, this time in mourning for the death of Eisenhower, March 30, 1969. Though she and Lee of course regretted the death of General Eisenhower, it did mean another $5,000 loss since Lee would have to continue paying the band under their contract during the downtime, and the shows lost from their calendar would never be rescheduled.

There was little to do in Da Nang. Lee did schedule free shows for the patients in the hospital on the first floor of their hotel. And they looked forward to the resumption of the shows.

Neither knew that meant even more trouble . . .

The next show was at Chu Lai. While the conditions there were no better than at Da Nang, Cristy did find that the troops were just as appreciative as elsewhere.

But Russell, her bandleader, was another matter.

She had barely finished singing her last number when Russell started packing up his equipment.

"He's just jealous, honey," Lee said after the show. "Look at the way he treats the soldiers whenever they talk to Flo. And just last week he told me he didn't think it was fair that you got all the applause. He says nobody appreciates him."

Just then Russell headed toward Cristy and Lee. His face was red, and it was obvious he was angry.

"I've had it, Lee!" he stormed. "I sing, and I lead the band, but Cristy takes all the bows. She's getting credit for what I do!"

"Now, wait a minute, Russell," Lee said. A crowd of GI's was gathering around them. "Let's talk about this later."

One of the GI's, a corporal Cristy and Lee knew as Jerry, walked up to Lee to whom he had talked all through Cristy's show. By his slurred speech it was obvious he was high on something.

"Yeah . . ." Jerry chimed in. "Let's talk about this later."

"No. I'm going to settle this right now, once and for all," Russell declared. He swung a meaty fist at Lee, caught him under the left eye, and sent him staggering. Lee lunged back at the big fatso, but a couple of soldiers stepped in and grabbed them both. However, Russell continued to rave at Lee and curse him.

Suddenly Jerry stepped in.

"That's it, man. No more." He stopped in front of Russell, pulled out his bayonet, and pointed the end of it at Russell's throat. "I've been watching you all evening, you fat pig. You're jealous of Cristy 'cause she's got talent and you ain't got nothing. I could see it." He jerked his head toward Lee. "Say the word, Lee, and I'll slice this pig's throat from ear to ear."

Russell was standing very still, his head tilted backward, his wide eyes staring at the glittering metal inches from his throat. Beads of sweat formed on his brow. Flo screamed.

"Don't do anything, Jerry. Please," Lee urged. "I can work it out with him."

"I want to kill him. He don't deserve to live. Either you or Cristy say the word, and I'll cut him wide open."

Cristy began to tremble. There was nothing anyone could do. Military police had moved in, but the bayonet was too close to Russell's throat for them to make a move.

"Please, somebody," Jerry snorted, "let me kill him."

"Don't do anything," Lee implored. "Put the bayonet down, please."

Jerry looked at Russell in contempt. "I guess they've saved your life, fat pig," he declared. His body weaved a bit, but the point of the bayonet kept its position. "You will apologize, though, or I'll kill you for myself."

Russell stammered, his voice weak. "I'm sorry, Cristy. I didn't mean it."

"Now apologize to Lee," Jerry urged.

"I . . . I'm sorry, Lee."

Jerry lowered the bayonet, and the police grabbed him instantly. The MP's turned to the crowd of soldiers and asked them what happened.

"The fat dude caused all the trouble," one soldier said.

"Yeah. You can't take Jerry," another added.

The tension among the soldiers was mounting. Lee said, "Sergeant, Jerry got a little carried away. Maybe a little too much booze. But nobody was hurt."

"I want to prefer charges!" Russell shouted, regaining his courage.

A tall, muscular corporal moved over to Russell. "Better think again, fat boy. Jerry wasn't the only one here who took a dislike to you over this."

"It's my troupe, sergeant," Lee said, "and I won't prefer charges." Then he turned to Russell. "As for you, you're fired! I want nothing more to do with you."

That night Cristy and Lee were given separate

quarters from the band until tempers cooled down. And the following morning at breakfast Lee told her he had made up his mind. He was going to cancel the rest of the tour.

Cristy knew the minute Lee walked into their hotel room in Saigon that the meeting with Tom Watchel, the Ladd Productions official, had not gone well. "He won't let us out of the contract. He said he'd sue us if we didn't finish the tour."

"Oh, no, Lee. What are we going to do?"

"It's either make up with Russell or hire a Vietnamese band—and you know how bad they are."

So, with the Ladd official acting as mediator between Lee and Russell, the thing was worked out as much as possible.

Then, in Can Thou, Cristy was too sick to go on stage. Wrapped in an Army blanket and shivering in spite of the 110-degree heat, she rode to the airport beside Lee. The Army doctor had said she should be taken back to Saigon and hospitalized. She was too sick to care . . .

But at the airport Lee was unable to get a flight back to Saigon. He pleaded. He stormed. He went all the way up the chain of command. He got nowhere. Until—

A stately-looking man in a business suit had been standing in the airport office by the window. He turned when he heard the commotion Lee was making and walked up to the colonel in charge.

"Maybe I can be of help. What's the problem?"

When the colonel explained the situation, the man said, matter-of-factly, "Well, my plane is ready to go. I think, under the circumstances, that I can make room for Mr. Stoller and his wife."

"That's not permitted, Mr. Winfield," the colonel answered. "Your plane is for cargo only and is not licensed to carry passengers. I cannot allow you to take them."

"Colonel," the man said calmly, "you sit here and play with your red tape. He says that's a sick woman over there. I'm leaving 300 pounds of cargo behind and taking the Stollers along with me. Have me cleared for takeoff . . ."

In Saigon the small white cubicle in which Cristy lay was like no other hospital room she had ever seen. It was large enough for one narrow bed and a dresser. There were no windows and no doors. Only a curtain separated her from the hallway where other patients were lined up in beds when the hospital was full.

"She has a virus of some kind," the doctor told Lee. "There are many viruses over here we don't even have a name for. But mainly your wife is suffering from diarrhea and malnutrition. We have got to get her fever under control and build her strength up. She'll be with us at least two weeks while we take x-rays and run tests. But the main thing is to build up her strength."

She was given antibiotics, tranquilizers, light nourishment—and the rest her body needed. She had lost 27 pounds, was down to a mere 74.

Meanwhile, Lee tried to salvage part of the show schedule by having the band fill the dates without Cristy. Russell enjoyed the spotlight tremendously. He sang and told stale jokes, but the soldiers' response was mediocre. There was no show without Cristy. After a few attempts, Lee cancelled the rest of the shows until Cristy was able to return.

At the end of two weeks Cristy had regained some of her lost weight and strength and was released from the hospital. They did shows for two days—then Paul became ill. Without him playing lead guitar the shows couldn't proceed, so Lee again had to cancel.

While waiting for Paul to recuperate, Cristy appeared on the military television program "Interlude," singing songs broadcast to the soldiers throughout Vietnam. An officer on the broadcast staff invited them out to dinner. They went to the International Club where they had their first American meal since leaving the States. The club, a VIP's-only organization, catered to wealthy business executives and high-ranking officers. Outsiders were allowed only as guests.

Paul came back to work after nine days. Lee figured illness had cost the troupe 23 days of shows. They completed the shows in the Saigon area and traveled to Pleiku for 12 more. A major approached Lee after one of the shows.

"Mr. Stoller, we have men up near the front who haven't had the chance to hear Cristy sing—or even see a show by anyone—in a good while. I wonder if you would consider letting Cristy fly up and visit them? It would certainly boost their morale."

"It's okay with me if it suits Cristy."

"However," the major continued, "there won't be room for you. And only two members of the band can go in the helicopter. I'll have to go since I'm flying the bird."

"What?" Cristy said. "Lee can't go?" *I've never done a show without Lee . . .*

"There just isn't room, Cristy. And he doesn't play an instrument."

"Lee, maybe it would be better if I didn't go."

"Major, would she be safe?"

"Oh, sure. We'll bring her back safe and sound in no time."

"Cristy, why don't you go? It would be a real treat for these boys to think you traveled all the way out to the jungle to see them."

"Well . . . if you really want me to . . ."

The major took her by the arm to lead her to the waiting helicopter. "Don't worry about a thing," he said over his shoulder to Lee. "She'll be fine."

I don't know about that, Cristy thought. Nervous, she clung to her seat tightly as the helicopter whirred over the rough terrain. Sitting so close to the wide-open sky in the bubble of the chopper was not her favorite way to fly . . .

She breathed a sigh of relief when they landed. But . . . Several bearded GI's seemed to climb out of the earth to help them disembark. Foxholes. So well-camouflaged she could not see them from where she stood. *What have I got myself into now?*

"Welcome to 'no man's land!' " one of the GI's shouted as the helicopter lifted off and she was left there. She turned to wave to the major as he piloted the helicopter up over the trees. He had promised to be back in an hour, but already Cristy wished that he was flying toward them instead of away.

The helicopter had just slipped beyond the trees out of sight when there was an explosion of gunfire and a ball of fire appeared where the whirring blades had just been.

Cristy jumped.

"You were lucky," the captain beside her said drily. "They could have shot it down on your way in."

There were feelings she had she could not put into words.

"He was coming back for you?" the captain asked.

"In an hour . . ."

"It may be tomorrow before they can send another chopper. Let me show you where you can go in case of emergency." He took her to a very deep

and very damp foxhole. Two wooden poles supported a camouflage sheet over it.

Cristy looked at him.

The captain, familiar with death and the unex-
pected, seemed to have a half smile on his face.

15

Y ou weren't serious about me staying here
overnight, were you?"

"I wanted you to be prepared. You never
can tell. It may take that long to get a chopper back
in here again for you. Come with me. I want you
to meet some of the troops."

Oh, if only Lee were with me . . . But she went with
the captain through the area, meeting the GI's and
shaking hands. Russell and Flo, though disoriented,
followed. Cristy sang a few songs for the men and
signed autographs. It was hard to concentrate,
knowing that the major she had just talked with an
hour ago was probably dead . . .

Two hours later a helicopter whirred over the
trees.

"There's your ride home," the captain said.

"But . . . I thought . . ."

"I was just kidding, Cristy. But, actually, you never can be too sure out here . . ."

Back in Pleiku, Lee was emphatic. "That's the last time you'll go anywhere without me. At least, if something happens, we'll be together."

She didn't argue.

For the next several days Cristy and Lee visited with the soldiers and walked the streets of Pleiku. They shopped in stores with dirt floors and bought strange, glittering objects of a different civilization.

"We may not take back much money, baby," Lee said. "But at least we have something for our folks to remember this country by."

They walked through the dirt streets in the staggering heat that hovered between 110 and 120 degrees. They saw naked children and half-naked adults roaming hopelessly the dirty avenues.

"It's too bad something can't be done to help them, Lee," Cristy said. "Surely America is sending money to feed these people. Where's it going?"

"Lining somebody's pockets," Lee remarked disgustedly. "The rake-off is unbelievable. I hadn't told you about it before, but one morning while you were at the hospital I walked in on a meeting at Ladd Productions between their officials and some South Vietnamese police. There must have been thousands of American dollars scattered all over a big conference table. The police were raking it into briefcase, suitcases—and even paper bags. Later Tom Watchell told me he had to cut the police in on what the service clubs paid in order to be allowed to operate in Vietnam."

"Why isn't something done about it?"

"Too many people in our country—people in high places—are in on the take. Remember the sergeant I went to see in Huntsville, Alabama about arranging for us to come to Vietnam?"

"Yes."

"Well, I read in the paper where he has been indicted for taking bribes and payoffs from service clubs while he was over here. They say he took hundreds of thousands of dollars."

"What will they do to him?"

"Probably a dishonorable discharge and a slap on the wrist. Corruption is so widespread that when someone is caught there is a rush to play it down because publicity at a trial might lead to people at the top."

She thought of the young sentry . . . even the major in the helicopter . . . "Our guys are fighting and dying for nothing . . ."

"Yes. This is a situation that will haunt our generation for years to come . . ."

They continued their shows in the Pleiku area, but now there was one welcome change. Instead of having to find food in the civilian sector they were now invited to eat in the mess halls with the soldiers. They stood in line with the fatigue-clad young men, holding their brightly-cleaned trays to receive portions of American-style food. For her especially it was a welcome change. And the GI's liked having a female in their presence. They competed to be able to sit beside her.

"Wait 'til my girl back home hears that I sat down and ate dinner with Cristy Lane," a Pfc from Oklahoma told her.

The friendliness of the soldiers toward her and their enthusiasm over her just being there helped to dispel some of the doubt she had over being in Vietnam.

One day the base commander called Lee and Cristy into his office. "You know," he said, "we feel very close to people like you and Cristy who are with the service clubs and are willing to come all the way out here to entertain us. I'm not knocking the USO. They do their job. But their entertainers never go anywhere near the fighting. I was just wondering if you would risk going a little farther to help us? It would mean a lot to my boys and me."

"How much farther?" Lee asked, and Cristy could tell by the apprehensive tone in his voice that he was thinking about her last ordeal.

"Well, we have men well back of the enemy lines. They've been there for months without relief. The danger and the tedium are hard on the morale. Would you consider letting us fly you back there for some brief appearances? I won't blame you if you say no. It is risky. We've asked other entertainers, but they have always refused."

"I don't know," Lee said. He looked at Cristy. "What do you think?"

Before she could answer, the officer interrupted. "I heard about the trouble you had before when the helicopter was shot down. This time we will give you an escort. You will be as safe as we can make it. But there is a definite danger. I want you to know that before you answer, one way or the other."

Cristy took Lee's hand and told the commander, "I'll go anywhere Lee goes."

Their band members refused, and it was Cristy and Lee who climbed into the helicopter dressed in helmets and flak jackets. She smiled at Lee. *He looks like a young boy in his helmet and flak jacket.* She looked down at her own jacket and straightened the heavy helmet she had been given. *I must look a little ridiculous myself . . .*

Flanked by two others, their helicopter flew over the jungle. She heard gunfire below her and was immediately thankful for the gear she had been told to wear. The helicopter on the right broke formation and attacked the position below, its rockets sending fiery trails of exploding destruction . . .

Cristy felt she was truly in the midst of the Vietnam War when they landed at Camp Oasis, the home for some 100 American boys in the Vietnamese wilderness. The tropical terrain showed the marks of fierce fighting. Foxholes were scattered around gun emplacements and command posts. Camouflage nets draped the ominously-huge barrels of the heavy artillery.

Cristy and Lee walked among the soldiers, shaking hands and signing autographs. She felt good inside. The GI's smiled and laughed with her. Their stubbly beards and embarrassed looks as she approached told her it had been a long time since they had been able to bathe, or sleep, or eat normally.

Cristy sang several songs for the men without accompaniment. Then a soldier brought out a weather-beaten guitar.

"Do you know this one, Cristy?" He began strumming and humming "Rose Garden." Cristy joined in. The soldier followed her throughout the camp as she took requests and played as Cristy sang. Lee had his camera and took pictures of Cristy with the GI's. One gunner asked her to pose with his artillery piece, and Cristy sat on the deadly steel barrel that seemed to reach into the horizon.

Later that evening, as Cristy and Lee sat talking with the camp's commanding officer, a runner approached.

"Sir, one of our forward patrols is requesting artillery support. All they need is your order to fire."

The commander reached for the telephone and began to smile. "Cristy, how about giving us a little help?"

"Sure."

He spoke into the phone. "Are the guns ready with the position?"

"Yessir."

"Stand by to fire. I'll have someone else give you the command." He handed the phone to Cristy. "Just say, 'Fire!'" he told her.

"Fire!" she said into the mouthpiece.

Nothing happened. There was silence. No sound of exploding artillery. Not even a reply over the phone.

"Fire!" Cristy repeated.

Still silence. The officer took the phone. "What's the problem, sergeant? Didn't you hear the order?"

"I heard a woman's voice, sir. I thought it was a VC trick."

The commander laughed. "That was Cristy Lane, the singer. She's visiting us."

"Cristy Lane! Hey, put her back on the line—sir."

Cristy took the phone. "Fire!" she repeated—and winced as the sound of gunfire exploded over the wire.

They flew back to Saigon June 1, 1969 after visiting several more camps behind the lines. Cristy was exhausted. Even the Park Hotel room that had seemed so disheartening on her arrival in Vietnam now looked like a castle. She longed for a good meal and a good night's sleep.

But the schedule kept her so busy performing in service clubs outside of Saigon that she had little time or opportunity for either. She noticed with dismay that she was losing weight again. Food and water seemed to be the biggest culprits.

"Baby, you don't look well," Lee told her after a show.

"I'm okay. We only have a few more weeks on the contract. And I don't want to let the guys down."

So they continued working the service clubs in the Saigon perimeter, always getting a good response, usually four ovations.

Then . . .

Cristy was doing a noon show, and again she had gotten four ovations. Waiting in the wings, preparing to walk back on stage for her encore, she suddenly felt dizzy. Her clothes stuck to her thin body, and cold beads of perspiration began to drip down the back of her neck. The humidity seemed worse than ever. She thought she would smother with the closeness. And her stomach . . . How could it be so sick with so little in it? Realizing how sick she was, she turned to Lee and gripped his arm.

"I don't think I can go back on. Everything's going 'round and 'round."

"That does it, honey. I'm cancelling the rest of

today's shows and taking you to the hospital. You're going to see a doctor."

It was the same thing. But this time the doctor took Lee aside. "You've got to get her away from this country, Lee. I want you to get her on the next flight to the U.S. I know you're both professional people and you want to keep your word on the shows over here, but I told Cristy and I'm telling you now, there are no drugs that can take the place of a proper diet and rest and relief from the tensions she's under. You can fly her home now, alive—or you can ship her home in a pine box later. That's the choice."

Even with Cristy's life on the line, Tom Watchell at Ladd Productions tried to hold Lee to the contract. It took hours for Lee to convince him that Russell and the band would stay. Even then Watchell tried to pay Lee less than agreed. It wasn't until Lee threatened to sue, that Watchell would settle— for some cash and a balance to be deposited in Lee's bank account in Peoria.

The last night in Saigon Cristy slept well for the first time in weeks, but a sleepless Lee sat at the dresser with a dim light burning and counted up the cost of the tour. In money, that is. The TET offensive cancellation, Eisenhower's death cancellation, Cristy's and Paul's illnesses had cost them a gross revenue loss of $28,900. His pencil scrawled across the paper. He looked at the painful figures. They had come to Vietnam, undergone the hardships and the dangers, risked Cristy's life. They had worked long hours under miserable conditions. And it had all been for nothing. There was no profit.

Their net *loss* was $12,500.

Cristy's deep breathing filled the room. Lee got up and walked to the window, looking out at the Saigon night. The rockets that by now were commonplace to him flashed across the sky. He shrugged his shoulders, forced a smile, and spoke softly to himself:

"We've been broke before . . . and came back . . ."

At least Cristy had brought joy to a lot of GI's.

The next morning, they boarded the plane for their long flight home, Cristy took her last look at the war torn country that had almost taken her life. The flight seemed endless, lasting close to 40 hours. But . . .

When the San Francisco skyline came up beneath the wing, Cristy said, "It's like heaven to be back in America." Although it was a hectic tour, the smiling faces and the compliments from the GI's had made it all worthwhile.

Lee was silent for a moment, then he said: "It may look silly, but you know what I'm going to do first, don't you?"

"Lee, you're not! . . . Are you?"

"Just watch me."

They were among the first to deplane.

Lee laughed merrily and knelt to kiss the ground in the midst of the scurrying feet.

16

Weeks after the joyful return to the children and Peoria, Cristy stood looking up at the new sign just erected on this old brownstone building in East Peoria. "Cristy's, Inc." She had mixed emotions. Here she was just back from Vietnam and already Lee was booking her at fairs and all the shows for his fund-raising projects. They hadn't even been home a month before he'd found this old club—"The Trade Winds"—and had made a down payment on it. Now she'd be working here every weekend.

She pushed open the door and wrinkled her nose. Lounges always had that same smell of stale smoke and old liquor in the daytime. She heard a strange creaking sound and looked over in its direction, but she was still blind from the sunlight outside.

"I think I hear you, but I can't see you," she called.

"I'm over here on the ladder," Lee's voice replied.

Cristy walked over to the far side of the lounge and looked up. Lee was stapling something to the ceiling. "What's that?"

"Insulation." He gave the staple gun one final jab and climbed down. "This place is going to sound great when I finish here. You're gonna love how your voice carries once you start singing, babe. It's all in the acoustics."

Cristy smiled. Lee Stoller never ceased to amaze her. As soon as they had returned from Vietnam he had gone to see Jerry Weistart, president of the Truitt Matthews Bank in Chillicothe and signed a $15,000 loan, placing a second mortgage on their house. He had hocked just about everything else they owned to pay off their debts. He had reassembled the group "The Misty Men" for her, and together they had played military bases as fast as he could book them. He had no intention of letting the momentum of their stint in Vietnam go to waste.

Today he looked tired. "Did you see the paper?"

"No. Why?"

"Well, you know how furious I was when the 1970 'Heart of Illinois Fair' wouldn't book you because they said you didn't have a big enough name?"

"Are you still upset about that, Lee? I thought we agreed to put it behind us."

"Let me read you what's in today's *Peoria Journal-Star*, a letter to the editor:

Why isn't Cristy Lane on the Fair bill? I would like to know why Cristy Lane is not appearing at the Heart of Illinois Fair in 1970. I was told by Cristy's manager that the Fair manager said no. I think this is a disgrace after she spent three months in Vietnam entertaining our young men. She not only came back broke, but almost lost her life over there. She was considered one of the very best entertainers to appear in Vietnam. A lot of other GI's like myself visited Miss Lane in the hospital. We know how sick she was. I know talent-wise there was no question, for she is great. And she's also a super person. She is scheduled for a lot of other fairs in 1970, but why not her home state fair? WE THE PEOPLE OF THIS ALL-AMERICAN CITY SHOULD PICKET THE HEART OF ILLINOIS FAIR IF CRISTY LANE IS NOT ON IT IN 1970.

A disgusted GI who spent a year in Vietnam.

"What do you think of that, Cristy?"

"I think it's a very nice letter, but I don't think it's going to change anything, Lee."

"Well, maybe not. But I'm glad it's there anyway. Just for the record." He folded the clipping and stuffed it into his pocket.

"How did your fund-raising meeting go this morning?"

"They wanted me to change the percentage around—to take 25 percent and give them 75 percent."

"So what did you tell them?"

"I told them it was fine with me. They could have the larger percentage as long as they paid expenses. I told them it would include the cost of phones, office space and staff to run the campaign, the sales commissions, printing of the program, the auditorium and its personnel, and the entertainment."

Cristy grinned. "And . . . ?"

"They thought about it. Then one person stood up and said he figured the original split was best. He said he'd heard that I do good work and that they would make a better profit with me than with any other promoter."

The lights in the dimly-lit lounge flickered off, then on, signalling closing time. Cristy was glad. It had been a long night, and she was ready to go home.

It had been a year and a half now since they returned from Vietnam, but it seemed to her that she had never really gotten over that trip, that she had been caught up in a continual whirlwind . . . like riding a roller coaster . . . When they weren't traveling on the road, with four musicians packed into their car and a trailer full of equipment behind, she was busy at "Cristy's, Inc."

She looked around for Lee. She wished he would hurry. She felt tired, awfully, awfully tired. *Did taking that extra Valium before I left home this evening have anything to do with it?* Maybe tonight she could get some sleep. The doctor said to take the Valium only when needed. *Well, lately I have needed them.* It seemed she could hardly sleep at all unless she took one or two. She sighed. *I feel like I did in the old days . . . before the Mayo Clinic . . .*

Lee was pushing again. Or, at least it seemed to her that he was. Partly it was his own project. He had been very upset about a deal with a rock group, "TW4." He and a friend, Don Chapman, had gone into partnership with a company called Brave Records and had agreed to record "TW4." The agreement had been with a handshake. Now "TW4" had changed their name to "STYX," gone with Wooden Nickel Records, and become a hot national act. And all Lee had was four of their songs signed to his publishing company, Harvey Wallbanger Music. No contract.

As for her, Lee wanted success for her so badly that it just wasn't happening fast enough for him. He had thought Vietnam would be a stepping stone in her career, but as it turned out people didn't even want to hear about it.

She looked back toward the bar. The soft pastel lights on the canopy seemed to blur together. *I must really be tired,* she thought. But she spotted Lee coming toward her.

"Are you okay?" he asked, looking at her strangely.

"Just fine. I want to go home . . ."

Sometime in the night Lee awoke with a start. The bathroom light was on, the door slightly ajar, and he thought he heard Cristy moan. He went for the door.

Cristy was leaning over the edge of the lavatory. Her knuckles were white from gripping the porcelain, and her face was ashen. Her eyes, looking at him through the mirror, seemed not to focus. He saw the bottle of nerve pills and asked, frightened: "Cristy! How many did you take?"

Her garbled response only frightened him more, so he guided her back to the bed and called the doctor.

After the vomiting and the black coffee she gave him a half-hearted smile. "I'm fine," she said. Her head was aching and her stomach was in knots. *But I'm really not fine . . .* she told herself.

The days began to run together for her. Sometimes she felt like Cristy Lane the singer, other days she was Ellie Johnston, a helpless little girl standing before a condemning preacher. She continued to take care of the house and the children. And she continued to sing at night to them and to read the

Bible. But deep in her heart she felt that she wasn't doing anything good enough.

One night, while she was getting ready to go to the club, she heard a piercing scream. Tammy had cut her chin and had to be taken to the hospital. A week later Kevin fell and broke his arm. And exactly another week later, Cindy, riding her bike, ran into a tree and broke her arm. The accidents added to the guilt Cristy already suffered from not being with her children enough due to her career. It pushed her to the edge.

When she wasn't singing at the club or on the road, Lee was taking her on occasional trips to Nashville to record—and to try and get her a recording contract. She shuddered every time she remembered one lecherous-eyed producer telling Lee, "Just leave the little lady with me for a few weeks. You go back to Peoria, and I'll make her a star."

She still had trouble getting to sleep at night. There always seemed to be too much to do and too little time to do it in. Worst of all, she didn't feel like she was pleasing anyone, not Lee—and especially not herself. But she kept the pressures all bottled up within her.

One Saturday afternoon she was sitting around the kitchen table at Charlie's house with her mother and her sister-in-law, Jackie, and she was unusually quiet. Charlie had returned from Vietnam, and Jackie was complaining about him. Jackie's voice droned on and on, and Cristy felt like something inside her was going to snap. Suddenly she knew she had to get out of the house.

"I've got to go," she said abruptly as she stood up.

"What do you mean?" Jackie said. "You just got here."

"I can't listen to any more of this. If something bothers you about Charlie, then why not tell him instead of us?" She turned to her mother. "Mom, I'll see you later."

She didn't wait for any response. She just picked up her purse and practically ran out the door. As she drove home she tried to hold back the tears that were beginning to blur her vision. She felt as if she would explode. When she finally did arrive at home she could not control herself any longer and began to cry hysterically.

Don, her drummer, who was baby-sitting, looked at her in alarm. "What's wrong, Cristy?"

"Get Lee! Get Lee!" she screamed . . . over and over . . .

Lee held her in his arms for hours as she cried uncontrollably. He didn't try to get her to explain herself. He simply stayed with her until her sobbing subsided.

Two days later he approached her on the subject of giving up singing. "Cristy, maybe we should forget about this music business. I've got my fundraising business going pretty well, and if you are this unhappy about singing, I think we ought to give it up before it's too late."

"I don't know, Lee. Maybe . . . Maybe that would be best."

"Fine. But for now you ought to get some rest."

For several days nothing was said by either about singing. It was Cristy who finally brought up the subject. "We've invested a lot of time and money in a singing career for me, haven't we, Lee?"

"Cristy, I have never for one moment wavered in my belief in your singing ability or that you could have a great future. The money and the time were well-invested. But your health is more important to me than all the records, all the fair dates, all the clubs."

She smiled and kissed him. "Thank you, sweetheart."

"I mean it, Cristy. I don't even want to think about your continuing to sing."

"But I do."

"What!"

"I've been doing a lot of thinking these past few days while I've relaxed around the house. Sure, you've put a lot into a career for me, and it has meant a great deal to you. But I've come to enjoy it, also. From time to time, that is. Maybe not always, because there's a lot of pressure on me when I perform. But there's a lot of pressure on you, too. We've made new friends. We've seen new places. Let's stick with it."

"But . . . Your health—"

"I think I can lick my health problems by myself without a lot of doctors and their prescriptions. I'll put my nerve pills aside. I'm going to watch my diet carefully and make sure I eat the right foods. I'm not going to let every little thing build up inside me. I've got to quit carrying everyone else's problems—especially my own family's—around on my shoulders. I want to go back to singing."

"Are you sure, honey?"

"Yes. Don't we still have some fair dates scheduled?"

"Several. I was going to cancel them."

"I want to do them. And . . . there's something else I've been thinking about . . ."

"What's that?"

"Would things go better if we moved away from here? Maybe to Nashville?"

She saw the grin start at the corners of Lee's lips and spread over his entire face.

"Honey," he said, "I've been thinking the same thing. I just never wanted to mention it."

17

C risty had made the decision to move to Nashville, yet—ironically—once there, the pace of their life was governed more by Lee's destiny than by hers. Happily, she watched him off as he drove to Nashville alone to find them a house. She could not at the time foresee what the future would bring.

They moved in the manner typical of Americans. On a September day in 1972 her brother Charlie's new pickup truck—with trailer attached—pulled up to the red brick ranch house on Apache Lane in Madison, Tennessee, a suburb of Nashville. She, Lee, and the children pulled up in the car behind Charlie.

The instant she saw it she knew she would like her new home. It had been built by a contractor for his own family—built well. It was convenient to schools and other facilities, and the other homes in the neighborhood were all new and neatly kept. Lee had chosen well. She laughed as she watched Tammy, Cindy, and Kevin darting in and out of the bedrooms. They like their new home, too.

"Look at this, Cristy," Lee said as he took her by the hand and led her to the lower level of the house. "I see this as our private living quarters as soon as we get settled in and can remodel it a little bit. Kind of like our own apartment."

She saw there was a fireplace in the bedroom. Cozy.

Lee pointed to a small room just off the main living room, his face beaming. "Even a little office right over there . . ."

While they were unloading, Lee filled her in on some of the details the move to Nashville would mean to him business-wise. Don Chapman, his partner in the Braves Record business, had moved to Nashville earlier and would share his office space with Lee.

"I'll just keep my fund-raising office in Peoria," Lee told Cristy. "Molly Goldsburgh there is very efficient and can handle things at that end. I'll use the long distance telephone to control it from here. I'll do most of my work out of the office with Don —splitting the rent. I can run up to Illinois for periodic checks—that sort of thing. And Frank Martin said he'd take me all over—even down to Texas—to meet more potential clients in the law enforcement field, for their fund-raising projects."

Frank Martin . . .

Cristy frowned.

She had doubts about Frank Martin, the chief deputy for the Madison County Sheriff's Office in Madison County, Illinois. [*What a coincidence!* she thought. *Madison County, Illinois . . . and now we're living in Madison, Tennessee . . .*] Maybe it was just a quirk of her mind, but there was just something about Frank Martin that she didn't like. *Premonition?* No. It couldn't be. Martin was the one who had introduced Lee to the Deputy Sheriff's Association which had turned into such a big fund-raising account for Lee. It was natural that he and Lee should become fast friends. Still . . .

"Hey! What's the matter?" Lee asked, reading the solemn look she had let come to her face.

"Oh . . . Nothing, really. You already know how I feel about Frank Martin." She shrugged. "It's just that I get a funny feeling whenever I talk to him. Call it a woman's intuition, but I just don't trust the man."

"That's because you don't know him, Cristy. He's a great guy. Really. It's thanks to him that I got the account for the Association this year."

Just then Charlie, unlocking the trailer, called: "Hey! I need a hand over here."

[But Lee did not hear. He was remembering how he had thought he had lost the account. Frank Martin had told him that Sheriff Patooney wanted to change the percentage at the last minute. He said Patooney didn't think it was fair that he didn't get anything out of it. It had been touchy, but Lee simply explained that he would give the usual 25 percent of the proceeds to the Association Director, and it was up to the Director to distribute as he saw fit . . .]

* * *

"Hey Cristy!" Charlie yelled. "Tell your husband to quit daydreaming. This thing's heavy."

Cristy turned and looked at her brother struggling with a large cardboard box. She smiled. *Good ol' Charlie!* He was always there when they needed him. *Gonna miss you, Charlie, when you're back in Illinois . . .*

Two months later the Stoller family had settled well into the routine of school and work, and weekends were fun times shared with friends. This particularly beautiful afternoon was no different. Cristy and Lee had just finished dinner with Don Chapman and his wife, Willie, when the phone rang.

It was Marty Jones, manager of Lee's club in Peoria.

"Charlie's been killed, Lee."

Only a mile from his home, in his truck, going around a sharp curve, he had hit a tree . . .

The shock of Charlie's death was a stunning blow for Cristy. That night, as she lay in bed, she thought her heart would break. The only person she had lost to whom she had been really close was her father. Now . . . Charlie was gone. He had been more than her brother; he was her best friend. She remembered with fondness how he used to sneak Cokes to her when she ran out at home . . . She remembered how happy she had been when he met them at the airport in Vietnam . . . how willing he had been to talk to her . . . or listen, when she needed an ear. She felt as though something special had gone out of her life.

Forever . . .

Meanwhile . . .

Lee was learning the inner workings of the music business in and around Nashville, but he also continued his fund-raising campaigns that now stretched from Illinois, Indiana, Iowa, Tennessee— all the way to Florida. His friendship with Frank Martin grew, and the deputy approached him with a new business venture. Martin had been moonlighting as a private detective and wanted to start his own company, "006." He needed $10,000 operating capital and would give Lee 50 percent of the company. Lee agreed, counting on Martin's experience to compensate for his own ignorance of the detective business. But he remained mostly in Nashville, flying out from time to time, Florida to Iowa, to check on his room managers at the fund-raising events.

But it was Cristy he had most at heart. He continued to cut regular recording sessions on her, investing the necessary $3,000 per session. He moved his and Don's office to 1201 16th Avenue South—in the heart of Nashville's fabled "Music Row"—and made the rounds of the major labels whenever he could find the time. He met with the expected rebuffs: "We're not signing any new artists right now . . . Our company has no need of any more female singers . . . The songs are good, but they don't show us anything new." The same answers over and over. But Lee was a salesman, and he was undaunted. Besides, he was very good at learning from experience. He came to the conclusion that, despite the number of executive headquarters in Nashville, the real final decisions were being made by higher-ups in Hollywood and New York. In time he learned he was probably right, that only a few people in the world of the "Major Labels" actually had authority to sign recording contracts or set up promotions for a new artist.

But if one were what is known in the Nashville trade as an "Independent Label" . . . He took his idea to Cristy.

"Baby, I've been to all the major labels, small labels, and producers I can find. It's a closed door. The only way we're going to get anywhere is to start our own independent label. I've got the cash flow from the fund-raising operations. We have the capital to risk. I may not know much about the record game, but I've forgotten more about business than most of these lazy jokers will ever know. I think I can develop new talent and handle promotions better than these jackasses who sit in their plush offices for just a couple of hours a day pushing buttons. They don't know what hard work is."

Cristy agreed . . .

* * *

But first there were loose ends that needed to be tied.

The detective agency he had started with Frank Martin foundered after a year—because Martin did not have enough time to devote to the business—and Lee suffered the loss. However, he and Frank Martin remained friends, Martin sometimes assisting him in fund-raising. A pleasant man in his mid-forties, Martin had the personality of a salesman, and he traveled with Lee a few times to introduce him to law agencies for fund-raising projects. Lee had obtained a letter of recommendation from the Madison County (Illinois) Sheriff, Maurice Patooney—as he had with every other organization he had done business with—so when he ventured as far as Texas, taking Frank Martin with him to a deputy sheriff's convention, he was able to make connections with several new clients in the Lone Star state. Also, Granite City, Illinois—which is in Madison County —had become an operations center for Lee in the Southern Illinois area. And Molly Goldsburgh, the secretary for the Madison County Deputy Sheriff's Association, was an asset to Lee in his work there.

As for Cristy, alone much of the time in Nashville, she wanted something to do. She had worked since she was a teen-ager. Now, with typesetting equipment Lee bought for her and had installed in their home, she did custom work for different printers, utilizing knowledge she had acquired at the printing company in Illinois where she had worked. But she missed singing. The occasional public appearances she was making were not enough.

"Lee, I wouldn't mind doing more fairs if you want me to. The money wouldn't hurt us any, would it?"

Lee laughed affectionately. "Money never hurts, baby. But I'm doing well enough in the fund-raising field."

"I know. I just thought I might help a little, maybe make a few more fair appearances. Don't you want to book me anymore?"

"Let's not talk about business tonight. I have a surprise for you. I'm taking my best girl out to a night club for dinner and dancing."

"Great. Where are we going?"

"To 'The Hearth'—the club we went to last weekend. I want to catch a new singer there."

They went, and the act, Daniel Willis, proved to be a super-talented young man. So, after the show, Lee invited him to come by his office and talk.

Lee now had a new office—at 120 Hickory Street in Madison, Tennessee—and a new company, "LS Records." He signed Daniel Willis to a contract. Cristy was enthusiastic about Daniel. The fund-raising projects were flourishing, and income from them would not only help pay for recording sessions, they also allowed Lee the opportunity to make other investments. He put $15,000 into a new photography business to operate from his office building and hired a professional photographer to run it. He borrowed another $10,000 and entered into a real estate sign-making business with Billy Arr, now in Nashville, and two other men.

Show dates were picking up for Cristy, and Lee bought a bus for her and the band to travel in. But . . . The bus proved to be a catastrophe. Major repairs, including a motor overhaul, were soon needed. Besides, it took a lot of cash to keep it on the road.

Then the investment in Daniel's career proved to be quite expensive. The records were barely charting.

The photography business failed.

So did the sign-making venture.

But the fund-raising business continued to prosper, and Cristy was recovering from her grief over Charlie's death. So the world looked bright . . . when the call came . . .

The Internal Revenue Service in Peoria. They wanted him to make an appointment to stop by their offices to answer some questions.

"Certainly," Lee said. "I'll come by the next time I'm in Peoria. Haven't I been paying enough taxes?"

"There are just a few questions we want to ask you, Mr. Stoller," the man said . . . coldly . . .

"Everything should be in order," Lee said.

"That's why I pay my accountants—to keep things in order."

"It won't take long—if you'll stop by our office at your earliest convenience."

Lee hung up the phone. His imagination mulled over the possibilities. What did they want? They had been auditing him ever since 1966—more than likely because he was self-employed and made a lot of money.

Like nearly all taxpaying American citizens who contend with the near-dictatorial powers of the Internal Revenue Service, Lee did not particularly look forward to his interview as he entered the IRS offices in Peoria. But he wasn't afraid; he paid his accountant handsomely to be certain his taxes were handled legally and properly.

"You have several different corporations, don't you, Mr. Stoller?"

"Yes, and each one pays its own taxes—as I do."

"I know," replied Shriker, who had introduced himself as a special investigator for the IRS. "This isn't a regular audit. We just want to clear up some things."

"Everything should be in order, Mr. Shriker. If something is wrong, I'll send my CPA down to talk to you."

"It doesn't work that way." Shriker drummed his pencil on the desk and continued to look steadily at Lee. "If your accountants make an error, whether intentionally or unintentionally, you are still liable

—even to the possibility of criminal prosecution."

"That doesn't sound quite fair. I have to rely on their integrity and accuracy."

"Mr. Stoller, if you put your name on the bottom of a tax form, the presumption is that you know what's there. As I said, though, this is not a regular audit. Tell me about the bus you bought."

Lee explained from memory the purchase cost and operational expenses of the bus he had bought for Cristy to tour in.

Shriker continued. "You list a loss of $10,000 for the '006' detective agency."

"Yes. I was in that with Frank Martin. It didn't work out. I documented my losses."

"You listed a $15,000 loss for the photography business."

"Yes. That didn't work out, either. I closed it down."

"What was this 'Back to the Soil' tax loss you listed?"

"In '75 I invested in a record album called 'Back to the Soil.' It was planned as a Bicentennial release honoring the American farmer. Grant Turner, the Grand Ole Opry announcer, narrated it. We tried to promote it through the Future Farmers of America. That also flopped. I lost about $10,000 on that."

Shriker went on to inquire about the sign business, then added: "You've had some substantial losses, Mr. Stoller, but your income gross continues to be substantial."

"I work hard." Lee smiled, trying to thaw the icy interview.

Shriker leaned forward, not smiling. "Cristy Lane, your wife, is a singer. Yet most of your income seems to come from fund-raising."

Lee nodded.

"You've handled fund drives for the Madison County Deputy Sheriff's Association?"

Lee thought it odd that Shriker should bring up just one association. "Up until a few years ago. They had a change in the Association officers, and the new officers didn't like the way the old ones disbursed the funds that had been raised. I told them I had nothing to do with the funds after I turned over the Association's percentage to them."

"Do you remember a man named Sam Stone?"

"Yes, vaguely. He was a sergeant with the Sheriff's department. And he was active in the Association."

"I have here a copy of a letter Mr. Stone wrote. Please look it over."

Lee took the letter. Addressed "To Whom It May Concern," the letter gave information about the Sheriff's Department being involved in extortion and bribery, soliciting money from houses of prostitution and towing services specifically. Lee's name was mentioned. The letter said Lee had paid extortion money to the sheriff to get a franchise on fund-raising for the Deputy Sheriff's Association. The writer concluded with a statement that he feared for his life because of the information he possessed.

"This is wild!" Lee said. He handed the letter back to Shriker. "Sounds like this man Stone has a wild imagination—or a screw loose."

"He left the letter with his girl friend for his own protection. She was afraid of getting involved. She turned it over to the FBI."

"I don't know anything about any of this," Lee said. "I have never paid the sheriff any money to do a fund-raising drive."

"No one has ever tried to get extra money out of you?" Shriker asked.

"Oh, I've sometimes had clients who wanted a bigger percentage. But when they saw the expense breakdown they also saw that I couldn't pay them any more than I do. My business is successful."

Shriker stood. "Thank you for coming, Mr. Stoller. We'll get back in touch with you if something else comes up."

The meeting disturbed Lee. Anything to do with the IRS ruffled him as it did most people. But he was mainly perplexed by the letter written by Stone. He just couldn't conceive of the businessmen he had known in The Deputy Sheriff's Association being involved in any such ventures. He called Frank Martin and told him of the meeting and of Stone's letter. Martin told him Stone was crazy, not to worry about it, it was nothing.

Lee decided to dismiss it from his mind and return to Nashville where there was someone more important to think about—

Cristy . . .

18

C risty put down her book. Usually there was nothing she liked better than to sit curled up in a big easy chair in her bedroom and read. But ever since Lee had told her about the IRS trouble she had been uneasy. Today she was even more restless than usual. She had an eerie feeling that something was going to happen today . . .

And yet . . .

Oddly, her intuition told her it might not necessarily be something bad . . . It might even be good . . .

She got up from the chair and looked tiredly at a box of reel-to-reel and cassette tapes waiting for her to wade through, searching for a song to record. She had had no idea how many new songs and new song ideas there were in this world. And Lee said he had only brought her a small percentage of the hundreds he received at the office!

She knelt down by the box and began to sort them out. Every day she would listen to several until she found one she liked well enough to record. Many times she would go through a whole stack and not find one, while on other days she found more than she and Lee could afford to cut.

Lee had already released three new records for her: "Midnight Blue," "Trying to Forget About You," and "Sweet Deceiver." How excited he had been each time! He would come home and say, "Honey, this is it! This one's gonna break it for us!" They hadn't, of course. They got some airplay and even made the national record charts which, Lee had explained, listed in the music trade magazines how popular a record was supposed to be. Actually, though, Lee hadn't done too badly for her. Each record had at least gone into the top 50. The trouble was, the cost had been staggering.

She wondered at times how Lee did all the things he did. He helped find songs for her. He was with her in the recording sessions. He was there for the mixdown . . . and the mastering . . . and the pressing of the record. And he saw to it that the releases were mailed to over 3,000 radio stations across the country. She tried to help as much as she could by going into the office part-time, helping with the printing of the flyers, the promotional posters, and the extensive mail-outs. In fact, she had just helped with the most expensive and ambitious mail-out yet, for her new single, "Let Me Down Easy." She had hopes for this one. It was from the 60's, and Lee had hired Charlie Black, an independent producer and songwriter, to produce the session on her. It was an uptempo song, and Lee was convinced it would be a hit.

Of course, she didn't want to get her hopes up too much. There had been too many disappointments before. But they had worked so long and hard, had spent so much money on her singing career, it seemed there ought to be some inevitable justice that would make it pay off. Besides, on this particular song Lee had signed with the GRT record label, a distributing company which would see that LS Records got to the record stores across the nation. Of course, if the records didn't sell, GRT would keep them unless Lee bought them back. But at least it was a large enough company to handle the job that was just too much for Lee's small staff. Maybe—

The front door slammed.

Suddenly she had a premonition that something was going to happen, and her heart came up into her throat.

"Cristy! Where are you?"

It was Lee's voice, and there was an unusual urgency in it. She looked at her watch. 11 A.M. He never came home this early. *Oh no!* she thought frantically, *what's gone wrong?*

"What in the world is the matter, Lee?"

He came into the room, and he was almost running. She looked at his face, trying to read the bad news in his eyes.

But he was beaming, beaming, beaming with joy.

He was holding a copy of *Billboard Magazine*, and he spread it out on the table with the flourish of a ringmaster at the circus. He didn't say anything at first, just pulled Cristy to him and kissed her. Then he announced, almost like a formal statement:

"It's been a long, hard climb, my dear. But— Look at this!"

Confused, Cristy scanned the page headed "Top 100 Country Singles." Under the Number 7 position Lee had drawn a red line. There was a black dot and the words: "Let Me Down Easy—Cristy Lane."

Now she understood.

"You've hit the top 10 of all the country songs in the nation! And you've got a bullet! Which means your record is still climbing!"

A warmness flooded over her.

After all the heartaches . . .

19

I got a letter from Chris Lane, the DJ. He's working at KGBS in Los Angeles now, and I asked him to write a few liner notes for your album cover. Want to hear what he wrote?"

"Of course."

Lee reached into his pocket and pulled out a slightly wrinkled sheet of typing paper. "He says that you have 'a woman-warm sound that leaves a cat paw gentleness in your ear.' He also says that he is very proud and honored that you are his namesake." He carefully folded the letter and kept on talking. "I'm getting calls from booking agents all over the country. One promoter even wanted to know who this 'Mystery Lady' was. He thought you were some background singer I had developed. Yeah, baby, pretty soon we'll be booking you for some real money."

But in the sunlit world of her coming success there was also the rising cloud of Lee's troubles with the IRS. Cristy asked Lee to explain to her what the latest problem was.

"It's pretty complicated, but the lawyers and accountants say it's legal. I've had to work some loans and property through the corporation, and some through my own name. At times I have borrowed money in my own name, using our personal property as collateral, and used the funds in the corporation. The government doesn't like that. They'd rather see cut-and-dry profits, that they can tax at the corporation rate and then tax again when the profits are paid out as dividends."

Despite his problems, Lee threw his total concentration into promoting Cristy's album—the album they had decided on when she hit big in the charts. The results were great, and Lee's scrapbook soon held such clippings as *Billboard*'s ". . . a Hit! 'Cristy Lane Is The Name' (the title of the album) is destined for the top." *Cashbox*'s "An excellent production brings Cristy Lane's soft and flowing voice up front. A pretty lady with a bright future." And *Record World* said that Cristy had a "tasteful style."

As the year neared a close, Cristy had placed four singles on the charts. She ranked in sales with artists the likes of Conway Twitty, Merle Haggard, and the Statler Brothers. Her position on the charts placed her ahead of such veterans as Barbara Mandrell, Ronnie Milsap, and Loretta Lynn.

Her career had finally taken off.

But Lee's problems worsened. In November he was summoned to appear before a Federal Grand Jury convening in Springfield, Illinois. Also summoned were his brother, Roy, and his campaign manager in Madison County, John Cornwell—as well as Frank Martin and others. Certain that he was innocent of wrongdoing, and trusting in the advice Martin's lawyer, Carl Brown, gave him, Lee took the Fifth Amendment and was excused. After it was over, Brown told him, "Go home and forget about this, Mr. Stoller. You've heard the last of it."

But Cristy felt differently. "You are too trusting, Lee. Maybe there's something going on in Madison County that you don't know about."

"I can't believe that. Frank is an honest man. He wouldn't do anything illegal—or be involved in extortion."

"I hope you're right, Lee."

"Well, the main thing is, I haven't done anything illegal. That crazy Stone said I paid the sheriff 10 percent to do business in Madison County. That's a lie. I give the Association 25 percent—and that's it. There isn't enough to pay any more. And, besides, the sheriff isn't even a member of the Association."

"I'm frightened, Lee," Cristy murmured. "I can't help it. I'm frightened."

"Don't be." He produced large sheets of hand-drawn graphs. "Here. Look how your latest record is climbing. I'm doing what *Billboard* and the trades do, charting your record myself with phone calls to the jocks. This new single is hot as a firecracker."

The name of her latest hit was . . . "I Just Can't Stay Married to You" . . .

* * *

Cristy tried to take Lee's advice about not worrying. After all, she had always left the decision-making to him—the big decisions, that is. But she couldn't help being worried. She knew Lee was a trusting person who stood by his friends. She had seen enough of the world to know that such blind loyalty could be disastrous.

The blow fell early in 1978. Lee was indicted for extortion and bribery along with the sheriff and the chief deputy. Lee was indicted under the RICO Act —which he had never heard of. He called his attorney for an explanation.

RICO stands for Racketeer Influenced and Corrupt Organizations, he was told. It was part of a series of laws passed in the early 1960s to attack organized crime, conspiracy laws whereby the government could prosecute persons for talking—or, supposedly, even *thinking*—about the commission of an illegal act, whether or not the party was involved. It had become Title 11 of the Organized Crime Control Act of 1970 and was originally implemented to give prosecutors more latitude in bringing criminal syndicates into court. However, the government soon found new uses for the act. When investigators lacked evidence linking certain suspects to a crime, the RICO Act was used to file conspiracy charges against individuals acquainted with the suspects—even though they themselves were remote from organized crime.

Lee immediately called Frank Martin. Again he got the "They have no case" advice, but this time Lee was adamant. He demanded to know why he was being dragged into all this.

Martin sighed. "My lawyer says the statute of limitations had run out on the charges they claimed against me and the sheriff back in the early 70s. To keep the case open, they had to link you to us in 1975 through the Madison County Deputy Sheriff's Association."

Lee was appalled. "You say I am being indicted just so they can get to you and the sheriff?"

"Yes. Otherwise, the time has run out, and they couldn't bring any charges to anyone."

"But, Frank, I had no idea you were ever involved in anything illegal."

"Who said I was, Lee? They're only charges. There is no proof."

"But . . . why me?"

"You're their link, Lee. They're claiming you bribed a public official, the sheriff, to do the fundraising in Madison County. By coming up with conspiracy charges against all three of us they can go back as far as they like to help build their case."

A stunned Lee Stoller continued the conversation . . . The charges were coming from Sam Stone because he had been caught and was trying to get out by implicating others . . . He was claiming that Lee had paid him and Martin 10 percent for the sheriff . . . Martin had arranged for a law-

yer for Lee. . . . The fee would be $5,000 . . . The
government was only trying to scare Lee—according to Martin . . .

"Trust me, Lee. You and I have been friends for
a long time. I won't let you down or steer you
wrong . . ."

But Cristy was not so sure. "I pray you are right,
Lee. Maybe he is your friend. But I know how
trusting you are with people. You believe the best
about everybody." *But I don't?* The thought was a
shock to her mind. Hadn't she always believed that
people were good? That the world was good? The
thoughts, the memories, the images began piling up
in her brain, rushing at her like the foreshortened
photography in a science fiction movie . . . triggered
by the blow of Lee's indictment.

If the government would callously and cruelly
use an innocent man for its own purposes, where
was justice?

Suddenly all the images and memories rushing at
her smashed into her mind . . . the cold voice of the
salesclerk who wouldn't hold the doll just a few
minutes for a single penny . . . the colder contempt
of the teacher over her polka dot dress . . . the
laughing face of the young machinegunner suddenly stilled . . . the death of the sentry . . . the cold
way the Ladd Productions official had taken advantage of them . . .

Was it really "God's beautiful world" . . . or a

wasteland where the brutal and the callous held sway? Mocking phrases clutched at her: "woman-warm voice with cat paw tenderness" . . . "sweetest voice this side of heaven" . . . She was a singer of sweet songs in a world of love and tenderness—but was it really that kind of world?

The thoughts, the images, the memories mixed in her mind, making no sense whatsoever . . . yet somehow covering some meaning she knew about deep within her—but could never share with Lee, now or ever. It hurt. Her voice had been level, but now it broke, and she began to cry even as she repeated: "You believe the best about everybody . . . but somehow I just don't trust Martin."

Not knowing what had been going through her mind, he pulled her to him. "Here, let me kiss away those tears. You know I wouldn't break the law. Nothing will happen to me."

But something did happen.

At the arraignment, the U. S. Attorney offered Lee immunity if he would plead guilty to tax evasion in one of the two counts against him. The other would be dropped, and Lee would be given probation. In return Lee was to furnish whatever information he had about corruption in Madison County.

Since he was not guilty of tax evasion, had broken no laws in Madison County, knew nothing of corruption there, and was certain his innocence would be vindicated, Lee refused. His new lawyer, Mike Costello—conflict of interest would not allow Brown to represent him—tried to get Lee's case tried separately. Judge Ackerman refused. He tried for a change of venue, but the sheriff refused. So Lee was to stand trial with the sheriff and with Frank Martin, the deputy, in the February term of court in Alton, Illinois, across the river from St. Louis.

Local media played up the role of the sheriff, who had been elected nine years earlier, but Lee's name got national recognition since he was Cristy Lane's husband and manager. Wire service and television reporters came to the trial because of Lee's connection.

And through it all, Lee tried to work on a "business-as-usual" basis. Cristy's song, "I Just Can't Stay Married to You," was leaping up in the charts, and Lee was throwing all his energy into promoting it—so much so that both Cristy and his attorney insisted Lee devote time to preparing for the trial.

Cristy could not hide her concern. "Lee, you're not taking this trial seriously enough."

"I'm innocent, honey. I know it. You know it. And the jury's bound to see it."

"I wish it were that simple. I'm afraid it won't be. I keep thinking: What if you have to go to prison? I can't stand that thought."

"Honey, I've never been in trouble with the law

in my life. Even if Frank and the sheriff are guilty, I've had nothing to do with the operations of the Madison County Sheriff's Office."

"Then why did they drag you into it?"

"Time has run out. The only way the government can get at Frank and the sheriff is through me. And, since I'm innocent, they'll have to throw the whole case out."

"I hope it's that easy."

"It will be. Don't worry. Hey! Your record is #1 in 20 markets across the country—and still spreading!" He smiled, mischievously. "I've been meaning to ask you, are you trying to tell me something with that song? That 'I Just Can't Stay Married to You?'"

"Lee! That's not funny!"

"Just joking, Cristy. Just joking." He put his hands on her shoulders and looked into her troubled eyes. "Now, come on, Cristy. Cheer up. It's not nearly as bad as you think. Let's just forget about it. Besides, I've got a surprise for you."

He walked over to his desk and proudly held up the finished album cover that had just come from the printer that day. "Your second album, baby— 'Love Lies.'"

Cristy sighed. She knew his mind was already miles away from the upcoming trial.

When the trial started Lee was so certain it would all be wrapped up in a hurry that he kept a phone nearby in the lawyers' conference room so that he could conduct business as usual.

But . . .

That first afternoon he sat in the courtroom and listened in startled interest as the story unfolded on the witness stand. He was glad that he had insisted Cristy stay home. She had been right about Martin all along. Lee couldn't believe his ears.

The prosecutor, through prompting his witnesses, brought out all the facts. The sheriff had taken office in Madison County in December, 1970 and had held the office until he was indicted by the Federal Grand Jury, November, 1978, leaving office the following month. It was brought out that, when the sheriff was inaugurated, deputies already on the force were taking bribes from towing services and houses of prostitution. But when the sheriff took office it was said that he changed the procedure so that payments would come directly to him instead of to the deputies. The sheriff's brother-in-law and a close friend were the two men who were to handle the transactions, but at Trick's Towing Service in Wood River, Illinois, one of their first visits, it was decided the brother-in-law lacked the tact needed for the job, so Frank Martin replaced him. They called on eleven establishments. Six agreed to the payoffs, and five refused for various reasons, one because he claimed he was already taking care of a judge in Madison County. Another red-light operation said that, while his bar was in Madison

County, the motel rooms where the prostitutes worked were in the rear of the bar which was legally in St. Claire County and therefore out of the sheriff's jurisdiction.

Witnesses revealed the system began to falter after the first year. A sergeant in the Sheriff's Office, unaware of the payoffs, ordered a raid on Myrene's Steak House, which was named as one of the principal contributors to the sheriff's organization. The sheriff made the sergeant promise never to call another raid without prior approval from the sheriff himself.

Then, two Assistant State's Attorneys, and, later, the State Police, had staged raids without telling the sheriff. During that raid, Club "J," an alleged house of prostitution, called the Sheriff's Office wanting to know why he was being raided. Evidence indicated that this club had paid the sheriff nearly $10,000 to guard against such raids.

The IRS entered the picture in 1974, investigating the sheriff's brother-in-law for the years 1970 through 1972. A story was concocted claiming the brother-in-law had been working for the sheriff undercover, and a dead man and a former deputy were blamed for the appropriations of illegal funds. But, under pressure, the brother-in-law had testified before the September, 1977 Federal Grand Jury and had told all he knew of the sheriff's operations. He was indicted and convicted of perjury and racketeering.

As the trial progressed, the government brought in witness after witness, day after day, to describe how they had made payoffs to the Sheriff's Office. Legal and illegal operations alike shared the witness stand. Lee sat through it all, unbelieving. When he reached the motel room he had rented for two weeks, he called Cristy.

"I don't understand why I'm here," he declared. "Neither do the newspaper and television people."

"When is it going to be over?" Cristy asked.

"Mike (Costello, Lee's lawyer) thinks another week. At the rate it's going, though, it seems like it will take another year. Every day, when the court adjourns, I feel like I've been back plowing all day in my father's soybean field. I'm exhausted from just sitting there."

"What happened to the man who wrote the letter, the one who made all those statements about your giving the sheriff money?"

"Haven't seen him. Don't worry, honey. Everything's going to be fine. Now, let me give you some good news. I've been charting your record from the courthouse during recess. It's doing great! I've made calls to . . ." He began reciting the names and call letters of radio stations. He was jubilant.

Cristy listened silently.

A sob hung in her throat . . .

20

*C*risty fought her strong desire to get on a
plane to be with Lee. Always before she
had needed him. Now she felt he needed
her, and she wanted to be by his side.

She followed the trial as best she could from the
media reports and Lee's telephone calls. This picture emerged:

During the second week of the trial the prosecution started the attack that apparently would strike
at Lee. It was shown that the Madison County Deputy Sheriff's Association, begun as a bargaining
unit for the law officers in 1970, became also a social
and charitable group, and in 1971, at the urging of
Frank Martin, Lee was contacted to organize and
promote a "Sheriffs' Dance" to raise money for the
DSA. Lee was to pay expenses and was to receive
75 percent of all proceeds, with 25 percent going to
the DSA.

Stone, called in from prison, claimed that after
the first month of solicitation for the dance, the
sheriff had called him and Martin into his office and
asked, "What's in it for Old John?" Stone claimed
Martin said he could work out something with
Stoller. His testimony was that they went together
to Lee, told him that without the sheriff's approval

any fund-raising activity was doomed. Stone stated that Lee at first objected to paying the sheriff 10 percent of the gross, but then agreed to it. Stone further stated that the DSA signed an exclusive contract with Lee and his corporation for future fund-raising, with Lee paying them for the sheriff. Stone claimed Lee paid $10,000 to $12,000, Stone and Martin skimming $3,000 for themselves.

In 1975, new officers for the DSA questioned the accounts, and there was a minor hitch concerning a check charged to the wrong account, but this was no big thing and was obviously a routine mistake.

Then Molly Goldsburgh, who had been both Lee's secretary and secretary for the DSA, was called to the stand. The federal prosecutor led her into an explanation of how funds were raised and how they were paid into the campaign headquarters. She said 40 percent of the funds came to the office in cash, a lie, and a dangerous one. (The actual percentage was around 5 percent.) Under cross-examination, Molly Goldsburgh repeated the figures—almost word for word as if memorized.

The way the trial was running had been too much for Cristy, and she had already come to a decision before Lee called that night after Molly's testimony. But his news shook her.

"Why would she say something to hurt you, Lee? Something that's not true?"

"I don't know. But I'm not worried about it. Mike is putting me on the stand tomorrow."

"Lee . . ." Cristy hesitated, then plunged on: "You may get mad at me for doing this, but I've made plane reservations for tonight. I'll be at the St. Louis airport three hours from now . . ."

Even sitting in the courtroom, Cristy still found the trial confusing. John Cornwell took the stand and testified that while he managed the DSA campaign not only had he not paid the sheriff any monies, to the best of his knowledge Lee had not, either. His testimony also refuted Molly's estimate of the percentage received in cash. Further, he testified that all monies were accounted for. Even IRS agents, placed on the stand, testified that the books balanced when they conducted their audit. The sheriff testified he had received no money from Lee —or anybody else. Martin did not take the stand.

Cristy watched anxiously as Lee took the stand. He told the court how his business was operated from initial contact with a client to final contribution settlement. He explained the 25 percent to the client, showing that sales commissions, printing, entertainment, and other expenses took about 60 percent of the gross, leaving him with approximately 15 percent.

On cross-examination, Lee was asked if he had ever paid any monies to Martin or Stone.

"Yes," he answered. There was a stir in the courtroom. Then Lee went on to explain that they had worked for his campaign headquarters and been paid like everybody else, and it was all documented in his records. He had signed receipts from them.

And, as to the 10 percent Stone claimed Lee had given for the sheriff, Lee stated emphatically that it was a lie, and that he had never paid the 10 percent Stone had claimed.

Back at the motel room, Cristy asked the lawyer what he thought, now that things were looking so good.

"I still feel confident we will win. The points of law favor us. Lee was never remotely involved in the alleged extortions in Madison County with the taverns and the houses of prostitution."

"Why is he here, then?"

"The RICO Act is pretty broad. The prosecution is claiming that Lee bribed public officials to give him a franchise in Madison County. They say this was part of an overall scheme and any monies paid Martin and the sheriff furthered an illegal operation."

"But what does it have to do with organized crime? That's what the RICO Act is all about, isn't it?" Cristy asked.

"This is a point that has to be tested in court. The government claims that federal law has been violated because the Sheriff's Office falls within the category of an enterprise being corrupted. This is still a question that hasn't been answered in court, if an elective office falls under RICO."

* * *

In the end it was that obscure point of law that
made all the difference. The impossible happened.
The verdict was "Guilty" . . .

Justice . . .

The word had a mocking sound in Cristy's
mind . . .

Lee's attorney told him he thought an appeals
court would set aside the verdict, but an appeal
could take from two to three years. Sentencing,
meanwhile, would come in about three months.
Lee and Cristy went home to Madison, Tennessee,
Lee trying to make up for lost time in promoting
Cristy's career.

He hesitated to tell her there were other problems. The company distributing their records,
GRT, was rumored to be in financial trouble. If
they were to go down, then all her records would
be tied up in the bankruptcy situation—unless he
bought them first. And that would take a great deal
of money. Money was now a problem. Although
the IRS had now abandoned their criminal claim
against him, the cost for tax attorneys and accountants had risen to over $35,000. GRT was overdue
$100,000 in payments for Cristy's record sales. His
creditors were beginning to call.

His total debt was now approximately $150,000.
But . . .

Cristy was being mentioned for one of the most

prestigious awards in country music. There was talk in the trade that she would be one of the five nominees for "Top New Female Vocalist" in the Academy of Country Music Awards for 1979.

It was only a dream . . .

But it was a dream almost within their grasp . . .

Maybe . . . Lee thought, *maybe the dream is here* . . .

21

I 've got some news for you," Lee said the moment he walked into the room. "You and I are flying out to Hollywood next week to talk to the people at GRT. I've just set it up with Larry Welk of GRT."

"Hollywood! I've always wanted to go there."

She was excited. Ever since she was a little girl just the name of the town had held a certain kind of wonder and magic. But she wasn't too excited to notice the mischievous glint in Lee's eyes. *He's got something else in mind, too* . . . she thought.

"We're going to Hollywood for another reason, too."

She waited, expectantly, not saying anything to spoil his sense of dramatic timing.

His voice was too-elaborately casual. "I got a phone call yesterday from The Academy of Country Music. You remember, I told you some of my disc jockey friends had said there was a rumor you might be nominated for 'The Top New Female Vocalist of the Year?' "

"Yes, I remember."

"You, my love, are one of the five singers nominated for 1979."

"Lee! You're kidding!"

"No. It's true. The Academy called and wanted to know if you would be available for the Awards Show May 2." He teased, "I think Harold and Tammy can handle the office if you think we can make it."

She smiled. "I think we can fit it in." She could tell by the look on Lee's face how proud he was. She was almost happier for him than for herself. *Of course I won't win . . . but just being nominated is an honor . . .*

Lee became serious. "I can see that you're not going to get your hopes up this time. I'm glad. Cristy, there's a lot of politicking that goes on at these awards. Major record companies and promotion people spend big bucks advertising—and long hours calling—to win these awards for their singers. They use block voting. They get a vote for every member of their staff, and they use these for the singer they are promoting. We're a small independent label. We don't have that size staff, and we don't have the money to do the promoting. To be honest, Cristy, I was so busy promoting your records I didn't even know the voting was coming up. I had completely forgotten about the awards."

"Who does the nominating and the voting?"

"The Academy is headquartered in Hollywood. That's where a lot of country music started—going back to 'The Singing Cowboys,' Gene Autry, Rex Allen. Anybody connected to country music— from singers to disc jockeys—can join, and each one has a vote. I never even thought about joining. It simply slipped my mind until the Academy called. I have to apologize to you in advance, honey. I know you're the greatest singer around, but I just haven't had the chance to tell enough people."

Cristy could tell that Lee was upset. It was obvious that he felt there was no way she could win and was blaming himself. *He needs me,* she thought, warmed again by this apparent reversal of their relationship. She put her arms around him.

"Lee, don't even think about that. Without your hard work—and faith in me—I wouldn't even have been nominated."

They kissed.

They needed each other . . .

* * *

In Hollywood, Lee went alone to discuss the
GRT problem with Larry Welk. Yes, bankruptcy
was inevitable. About the two dozen songs and
two albums of Cristy's GRT held . . . Yes, GRT
would sell the stock and the albums back to Lee,
which would avoid the merchandise being im-
pounded by a bankruptcy court with resultant disastrous consequences for Cristy's career. GRT
also gave Lee a settlement from the company for
some of the expenses Lee had incurred. It would
help.

But he would still suffer a loss of over $100,000 . . .

On the ride back to the hotel, Lee decided not to
tell Cristy the extent of their losses.

For Cristy, the next five days were a whirlwind
of activity. She appeared with baseball pitcher Don
Drysdale during a broadcast of the game between
the Angels and the Red Sox at Anaheim Stadium.
She and Lee dined at famous restaurants. She was
thrilled when she spotted Clint Eastwood at a table
across from theirs in Alan Hale's restaurant. She
had grown up in an age when young girls idolized
movie stars, and this was like a childhood fantasy
come true.

She appeared on the Merv Griffin Show, then
the Dinah Shore Show. Dinah, she discovered,
was as relaxed and easy-going in person as on TV,
and it was this that helped calm Cristy's nerves,

jumpy at the very thought of being interviewed on nationwide television by such a celebrity as Dinah Shore.

It never crossed Cristy's mind that she was becoming a celebrity in her own right. Back home in Nashville, after Cristy's name and photograph had appeared on the covers of trade publications and in newspapers, strangers had stopped her in the grocery store or at a shopping mall and asked her for an autograph, and she had not seen it as the first step in celebrity status. Then she had been just a little embarrassed—but secretly thrilled—because inside she was still the shy little girl from East Peoria, Illinois. Now it was no different. It never once occurred to her that her's was an exciting story—that of the small-town girl who had achieved stardom on her own independent label started by her husband. Even after rehearsal for the Awards show she approached the event as fun. She never once entertained the idea she could win . . .

Once seated, Cristy looked around at their guests. Lee had made reservations for a party of ten at one of the front tables reserved for the nominees, and these were old friends for the most part. Chris Lane and his wife, Cherie, were there. He had moved from Chicago and was now one of the leading radio personalities in the nation. There was "Uncle Fred" Benson, one of the first promotion men Lee had hired to plug Cristy's records on the West Coast. With him was Red Doff, the public relations man he had recommended to Lee. Cathy Hahn, music director of KLAC in Los Angeles, and Don Langford, also of KLAC, were there, as were Ron West, program director of KSON in San Diego, and Mike Larson, formerly of Chicago and Lee's friend for over 10 years, and now with KSON.

Her gaze moved from her table to the crowded room. Suddenly she caught her breath as a lady in a simple flared western dress walked by . . . a polka dot dress . . .

Why should that bother me now? I ought to laugh at myself, she thought. It had been years since that night when as a high school girl she had been humiliated, yet she could still see in her mind the red velvet drapes of the school auditorium . . . the sharp, beak-nosed face of the cold-eyed teacher . . . could still taste in her mouth the bitter salt of her own tears . . .

Once again, I'm up for somebody's approval . . . or disapproval . . . Maybe the polka dot dress was an omen, a portent, a sign to tell her in advance that she was not going to win. That she would come close . . . like the single penny for the doll . . . like the tour of Vietnam . . . like—

But she already knew she wasn't going to win, so it no longer mattered. She breathed a sigh of relief. Tonight she had nothing to worry about. Tonight she was simply going to enjoy herself.

* * *

The actual award ceremony was easy on Cristy. She sang a segment of her current hit, "Simple Little Words," and then stepped back in line with the other contestants—Susie Allanson, Zela Lehr, Charly McClain, and Bonnie Tyler. She waited while each sang a portion of their own presently-popular songs. She could relax now. Her part was over. It was very pleasant not being under pressure, and she was enjoying every minute of it.

Dennis Weaver, Barbara Mandrell, and Roy Clark were co-hosts for the entire Awards Show, but for the segment, "The Top New Female Vocalist," it was the duty of Conway Twitty and Donna Fargo to announce the nominees—and the winner.

When the final vocalist had finished her portion of her own hit, the camera swung to Conway and Donna. Conway opened the envelope containing the name of the winner. He smiled and handed the paper to Donna Fargo.

"I'll give you the pleasure of announcing this winner, Donna."

Cristy smiled and looked toward Susie Allanson who had leaned forward now in anticipation.

In her usual robust style, Donna Fargo announced:

"The winner is—"

22

*T*ammy, Cindy, and Kevin, at home in Tennessee, had decided not to watch the awards. Fate had done a number on Mom too many times in the past. They didn't want to see this one.

But at the last minute Tammy's boyfriend just happened to click the TV switch while Tammy was walking into the den with a bowl of popcorn. It was just in time to catch Cristy singing the segment of "Simple Little Words." The TV stayed on through the presentation of the other contestants, but when it came time for the actual award, when Conway Twitty handed the name to Donna Fargo, Tammy got up to change channels. Her hand was just about to touch the channel selector when Donna Fargo's booming voice proclaimed:

"The winner is—Cristy Lane!"

Tammy squealed with delight.

The camera swung to Cristy then, and Tammy saw the evident shock on her mother's face, the stunned, I-don't-believe-it expression in her eyes . . .

Cristy couldn't move. It must be a dream . . . But the wild roar of applause and "Simple Little

Words" playing in the background convinced her. She started for the rostrum. It looked like it was a mile away. The TV cameras followed her every step. The room wavered before her, and she realized her eyes were washed with tears.

When she was on the rostrum it was all confusion. Donna Fargo and Conway Twitty hugged her. The big 18-inch silver-plated trophy was in her arms, the western hat that topped it scraping her ear. She stood bathed in the spotlight, and outside it the press cameras flashed. She found it hard to speak. Her voice was choked with emotion.

"Thank you all. I did not expect to win this honor. I am very grateful for it. There's one person I want to thank—my husband, Lee Stoller. Lee, stand up and take a bow. This—" She held up the trophy. "—is for you."

Lee's table had gone wild from the very moment her name had been called. They still were, and when the camera found the table, Lee and Chris Lane were both on their feet, shouting and applauding.

Cristy was still in a daze when Lee and Red Doff led her to the large room set up for media interviews. She answered the TV and radio reporters as though she were in a dream.

But a good dream . . .

Later, much later, when it was all over, and she was lying in bed with Lee in the dark, he said, "It's been a rough road to get here, baby. We've been through a lot together."

She rolled over on her side to face him. "That trophy should have had your name on it as well as mine. We're here because of you. My singing has always been for you."

"The award is all yours, Cristy. Chris Lane said something while you were in the media room about going to award parties for 30 years and of all the winners he had ever known, none deserved it more than you. It's all yours, Cristy. Your voice got you here."

"It took more than a voice, Lee. Your faith and perseverance did it." She reached for him in the dark and kissed him softly. It was the happiest night of her life. Winning the award had helped dispel that nagging sense of worthlessness that had plagued her ever since she was a child. Now . . . God had been good to her today. Silently in her mind she repeated the Lord's Prayer and then added, again silently, *Thank You, Sweet Jesus . . .* and drifted into a deep and peaceful sleep.

Lee lay wide-a-wake as he listened to the rhythmic breathing of his wife. He had done some figuring while Cristy was being interviewed. After all the work and sacrifice they had now reached the pinnacle of success. Cristy had the highest honor a newcomer in country music could receive.

But . . .

They were near bankruptcy.

He was free from GRT, but now he had lost his distributor, and he knew that an independent label without a distributor was hopeless.

But there was a bright spot on the horizon . . . the possibility of Cristy going with a major label.

The next day Lee talked with the owners of General Talent in Hollywood and signed them as Cristy's agent.

So when they headed back to Nashville he was optimistic once again. Back home they enjoyed more acclaim from friends and congratulations from family—and Lee was besieged with requests for appearances by Cristy. He could be selective now, and he wanted to choose carefully.

Oddly, the first appearance he chose for her after the Awards Show was a free one—at the Jimmie Rodgers Festival in Meridian, Mississippi. There was a certain appropriateness. Jimmie Rodgers, one of the founding stars of country music, had, like Cristy, bucked the odds. Brought up in a section of Meridian that was probably even poorer than the East Peoria Cristy had known as a child, Jimmie Rodgers had, like Lee, worked for a railroad, in Rodgers' case the New Orleans and Northeastern, a part of the Southern system. He had ridden many a weary mile in a wooden caboose before his unique style of yodelling had been cut by RCA. Whether Lee thought of all the similarities or not, he never told Cristy. But the festival was important. It was held each year, and it featured stars like Merle Haggard and Marty Robbins.

For Cristy, it was her first appearance with her new Nashville road band. Lee had put the band together. There was Quentin Good, affectionately known as "Big Q" because of his size and weight, who had been one of the original "Misty Men" at "Cristy's, Inc." as bass player. Mike "The Kid" Shannon of Flat River, Missouri would play saxophone, clarinet, and flute. Jim Wolfe was the drummer, Robert "Flames" Thames the guitarist, Chapin Hartford and Jim Foster the background singers, and Bill Wence the pianist and bandleader.

Lee drove the bus, and Cristy loved her private room at the rear of the bus with its blue-and-white carpet, curtains, and comfortable couch that pulled out to a double bed. But it relaxed her to sit up front and watch Lee drive.

It turned out to be a great way to start a summer tour. The auditorium was packed, and the crowd gave her a standing ovation when she finished singing her last song, "Simple Little Words."

Everything was perfect . . . except . . .

That today was May 14 . . .

And Lee's date for sentencing was only eleven days away . . .

* * *

On May 25, Cristy sat near Lee in the court-room.

The judge entered.

The U. S. Attorney asked for a 15-year sentence for Lee and a $50,000 fine against his company.

The judge shook his head. He said a 15-year sentence would be ridiculous. "I really have trouble, Mr. Stoller, in imposing a three-year sentence on you at this time, but that is what I am going to order. I want to review your case after your appeals, before you go off, but as of now I am imposing a three-year sentence."

The words hit Cristy like a fist.

But when she got back to Nashville with Lee there was a message waiting for Lee. He was to call Jim Golden of General Talent. The news was good, very good. Every major label in Hollywood wanted to sign Cristy, but Golden felt United Artists was the best. They were one of the largest, the money they talked was good, and they agreed to spend a lot promoting Cristy.

Naturally they flew to Hollywood.

Cristy and Lee and their agents sat before the imposing desk of United Artists' executive vice-president, Don Grierson. "We consider you an exceptional talent," Don said to her. "Your style appeals to the masses. We are not looking at one or two records, but many releases. If the first or second one doesn't hit the top of the charts, we won't worry because we know there is a future in your voice. We expect a very successful long-term working relationship with you."

The contract they handed Lee was 44 pages long, but it was a good contract. It would bring Cristy and him the much-needed cash he sought to pay his patient creditors. The four-and-a-half year agreement gave attractive royalties and promised considerable investments for promotion. United Artists agreed to carry the "LS" logo on Cristy's records, and they would buy up all existing masters from GRT.

Cristy listened as Lee and Don discussed the release of her first album with the company. It was decided to pull some songs already cut off the GRT album "Love Lies," record some new songs, and package the combination in an album called "Simple Little Words."

So . . .

Two weeks later Cristy saw the tangible results of that meeting in the January 23, 1979 issue of *Record World*, the influential music industry trade publication. There was a picture of her with Lee, Don Grierson, and Jim Mazza, president of EMI /UA. And the byline announced to all the industry that Cristy Lane had signed with United Artists Records.

She had arrived.

The outsider on the independent label, the little girl from East Peoria, had joined the club of successful country music stars.

* * *

But destiny, providence . . . God . . . had one more thing in mind for Cristy Lane, and a show in Evansville, Indiana, appropriately in the heartland of America, started it all.

Since signing with United Artists, Cristy had continued to tour regularly, but she was particularly excited about tonight's show in Evansville. It would be the first time that she would close her performance with a song that had come to mean a great deal to her.

Her life had been a roller coaster of joy and sorrow, and many times she had wondered how she would make it through the next day. There were times when she had needed a strength from beyond herself . . . *Please, sweet Jesus, help me* . . .—And He had, for her faith had been deeply rooted in her since her childhood, and she had been saved when she and Carol Hatcher had gone to Sunday services together. That had been a long time ago. She had called on God many times since then: . . . searching for a sense of true worth in herself . . . getting over her terror of singing before an audience . . . finding the strength to handle the loneliness and fear during Lee's trial and sentencing.

Yet that was all inward, private between her and God. She would like to express to others—but she didn't know how—the way she really felt. Now she had finally found one song that could do it for her. The lyrics summed up her life—and how, over the years, she had learned to live it. "One Day at a Time" would be her testimony. She had known the song would be perfect for her from the day Lee brought a copy home—known it even before she knew the history of the song itself. "One Day at a Time" was itself the testimony of Marijohn Wilkin in her battle against alcoholism, and its lyrics were born of Marijohn's own deep emotional struggle. But the co-writer was Kris Kristofferson, so it combined the best of two worlds.

That evening Cristy did close her show with "One Day at a Time" . . . and she found a closeness with the audience and a warmth she had not known before. For the first time she felt that she was sharing an important part of herself with her listeners.

But she was not prepared for how they felt until after the show when the crowd gave her a standing ovation, then gathered around her to talk and shake her hand.

"I love 'One Day at a Time,' Cristy," one woman said as she held out her program for an autograph. "When you sing it, I feel like it's coming straight from your heart—like you believe every word you're singing."

Cristy smiled. "That's because I do."

Young and old alike came up to Cristy that night. Some even wanted to tell her their whole life stories and why "One Day at a Time" meant so much to them. Others simply wanted to thank her for helping them feel better just for one night about a personal sadness they were experiencing.

Nothing like this had ever happened to Cristy before.

She turned toward Lee, watching from the edge of the crowd.

There was an odd look on his face.

She wondered what he was thinking . . .

Lee had felt the magic when Cristy sang the song.

But he was amazed at the reaction.

He had never seen any audience so enthusiastic over anything else Cristy had sung before . . .

The idea began forming in his mind . . .

Almost as though he were being led by some Power beyond himself . . .

23

"You have got to be kidding!"

Jerry Seabolt, Nashville based promotions man for United Artists, had that I-can't-believe-my-ears look on his face. He exploded into laughter, derisive laughter. " 'One Day at a Time?' Lee, you're putting me on."

Cristy and Lee were sitting in the United Artists office in Nashville with Seabolt, Jerry Gillespie, and Don Grierson planning Cristy's second UA album, "Ask Me to Dance." Lee had just suggested releasing "One Day at a Time" as Cristy's next single. Neither was prepared for Seabolt's outburst. Their faces must have showed it because Jerry began to explain patiently:

"Lee, that song has never been a hit. It was written almost 10 years ago, has been recorded by over 200 artists—and it has never made an impression on the public. Even some of the greats in the gospel field have cut it. Zilch! It would be a big mistake for Cristy. We don't want her to record a dud and release it to the public. It's not new. The jocks won't cooperate. You can bet on that."

"I know promotion might not be easy at first," Lee answered. "But I know it will be a hit if we can get people to just listen to the words. I think it could be a smash. And besides, it means something special to Cristy."

Don Grierson had not said a word. Lee looked at him. It was Grierson who had the power.

Don leaned back in his chair, thought a moment, then got up slowly. "Lee," he said softly, "so far you have picked six consecutive hits for Cristy. That's a very, very good track record. I'm going to leave this decision up to you. Whatever you decide, UA will back you up."

One week later, Cristy walked into the studio. *It should be easy today,* she thought. The musicians had already recorded the music, and she had sung along to familiarize them with the melody. But now she was going to put her final vocal on the tracks. What she sang today listeners all over the world would be hearing.

Cristy walked over and dimmed the lights. She smiled, remembering how difficult an act as simple as that had been when she first started recording. The musicians, too—she had always been nervous with them around, intimidated, fearful she would make a mistake and be embarrassed by it in front of them. *I've "come a long way, baby,"* she thought, self-amused. She had learned to block everyone else around her out of her mind when she sang. She would adjust her headsets and pretend she was all alone . . . alone with the lyrics of the song . . .

But today she was slightly nervous for a different reason entirely. She wanted this recording to be just right. For reasons deep within her mind, reasons not clear to her, it had to be "just right" . . . She stepped up to the microphone and waited while the engineer adjusted the levels in the control room. Just before the tape started rolling she did the one thing she had learned to do before every performance and before every recording session; silently, she recited The Lord's Prayer . . . *Our Father, who art in heaven . . .*

When the music began, Cristy sang, sang as she had never sung before. Pictures formed in her mind . . . a frightened schoolgirl standing before a preacher . . . a heartbroken sophomore turned away because of her dress . . . that early terror of singing before an audience . . . the horror of Vietnam . . . but, Lee's love and encouragement . . . and the slow climb to success . . . and when she got to "Sweet Jesus," in her own mind it became a personal prayer for the courage to face the three-year prison term hanging over Lee . . .

Afterwards, in the control room, she listened intently as the recording was played back. Usually she couldn't tell whether she liked the way she had sung a song or not.

This time it was different.

Today she smiled.

She liked what she heard . . .

Lee sat in his office studying the tracking sheet he was keeping on Cristy's "One Day at a Time." It had just been released, and it was getting off to a slow start. He was putting all his effort into promoting the record in spite of the resistance he was getting from disc jockeys and music directors. Before they listened to it they tagged it as "too old" or "too religious" for a country station. He did not want to admit that Siebolt had been right. But—

"Dad, are you real busy?" Tammy leaned around the open door. Tammy worked as Lee's private secretary and had become a strong asset to his operation. "Dave Segal is on the phone from Columbus, Ohio. Do you have time to talk to him?"

Lee liked Dave, a hard worker with 20 years' experience in the music business. But he was not prepared for the explosive voice that came to him over the phone.

"Lee, Cristy has an absolute smash! I've been listening to it all day! I had stations here ask why you released that song by Cristy when so many had recorded it before her, and I'm telling them all the same thing: 'Listen to it! Listen to the way she sings that song—and the way she says "Sweet Jesus." ' I tell them it's going to be the greatest record of all time. Lee, put the record on your stereo in your office and hear the way Cristy says 'Sweet Jesus.' "

Lee laughed. "You don't have to sell me, Dave. I've heard it many times. I know it's a great song and that Cristy sings it best."

"But you've got to hear it again—for me!"

"Dave, I tell you, I've heard it."

"Play it for me, Lee. Listen to the way she says it. Cristy really feels that song. I'm not going to get off the phone until you play it—and listen to those two words especially."

Lee put the receiver down and played the song while Dave waited.

"You're right," Lee acknowledged. "I never really thought about those two words. There is emphasis on them—a special feeling."

"This record is going to surprise even you," Dave said. "It's going to reach beyond your wildest dreams."

Lee, known as promotion man Jack Andrews to the jocks, was constantly on the phone to the radio stations, while Tammy and Harold called the stores.

Little by little music directors reluctantly slipped the song into their playlist. Disc jockeys who avoided the song began to get calls requesting it. Slowly, but surely, the record took off and began climbing the charts.

Fifty major markets showed that it was their number one seller. "The Record Center" in Cleveland sold the record so fast that they ordered this single by the boxes, 100 records in each, and still it was in such demand that a box was kept handy by the cash register.

There were some problems. Some stations gave it limited play—or no airtime at all. And at one point *Record World* dropped the bullet because the chart director "felt certain the record would soon fade away." It didn't. Even *Billboard* thought it would slip. But then *Billboard* was forced to jump the record from the number four spot where it had been for three weeks, to number one in the nation—over such dynamic artists as Don Williams and Kenny

Rogers. They had no choice; of the one hundred and some stations polled by *Billboard*, "One Day at a Time" was number one on 97 of them, and the number one selling record across the nation.

United Artists ran a front page ad in *Billboard* March 1, 1980. Part of the copy read: "CRISTY LANE—Fast becoming one of the hottest names in Country. With all the turmoil in the world today, perhaps the answer lies within her new single, 'One Day at a Time.' From her forthcoming album, 'Ask Me to Dance.' On United Artists records and tapes. (LT-1023)."

And Cristy received this telegram: "It's one thing to have a hit, but there's nothing better than number one—and the best is yet to come! Congratulations!" It was signed, "Jim Mazza, President, United Artists Records."

The Juke Box Programmer, a tabulation of what the coin machine operators wanted for their customers, ranked "One Day at a Time" in first place.

The people wanted to hear it, paid their money to play it, and bought copies to own it.

But Lee was still not satisfied. He tried K-Mart, J. C. Penney, Sears. But the rack dealers who had franchises in these stores had limited space to stock records and little faith in country or gospel songs.

So he came up with another plan. He told Don Grierson, "I have an idea that would sell half a million albums of Cristy's songs."

"Let's hear it."

"Advertise on TV."

"Forget it, Lee."

"Why?"

"It sells soap, cars, and most everything else you can think of. But it hasn't been that successful with records. Over 75 percent of all television albums fail. Some of the top superstars have tried it—and fallen flat on their faces."

But several weeks later Lee found the solution to the problem of TV sales. The Suffolk Marketing firm was so excited about doing an exclusive album on Cristy that they offered to order 20,000 albums in advance. *That* got Don Grierson's immediate attention.

Still, though, there was a problem.

Cristy didn't feel right about making money off gospel songs, and it was not until Lee pointed out how much the song meant to those who heard it, when he put it on the basis of actual effect this testimony in song would have, she listened. Even then, though, if she hadn't been allowed to pick all 18 gospel songs that went into the album, it might have been another story. As it finally came out, the album was her true testimony, out of the depths of her experience and being . . . for she, too, with God's help . . . had lived one day at a time . . . and would continue to do so . . .

*   *   *

Cristy filmed the commercial for the advertising campaign at the Grand Ole Opry House in Nashville. Television advertising began at the end of February, 1981, and ads were placed in publications with a circulation of 4,000,000 or more—*TV Guide*, *Parade*, *Family Weekly*, *Good Housekeeping*, *Woman's Day*, *Aarp*, *Grit*, *Elks*, and others.

From the very beginning, the campaign was a success.

Within a matter of months *over a half million albums were sold!* And that was only the beginning. K-Tel sold the album in Canada. EMI offered it in New Zealand and Australia.

The little girl who had once hidden behind a curtain at a Sunday church service to sing now had the number one country and gospel song—

Not only in her own United States—

But number one in all God's big beautiful world!

24

The sporty '73 Mercedes 450SL came to a stop at the corner of Gallatin Road and Neely's Bend. Cristy sat comfortably behind the driver's seat and adjusted her dark sunglasses. Her eyes were so sensitive that the thought of walking outside without them made her wince.

"You hoo! Excuse me."

Cristy turned her head and saw a lady in the car next to her waving her hands frantically trying to get her attention.

"Aren't you Cristy Lane?" she practically shouted above the surrounding traffic.

Cristy smiled and nodded, still unaccustomed to the increased recognition she received since the TV album had been released.

"I just bought your album and I love it," the lady chatted enthusiastically. "Could I have your autograph?" She thrust a crumpled piece of paper and a pen in Cristy's direction through the open car window.

Cristy looked around her anxiously. She hated to say no but she didn't want to hold up traffic either. There were no cars behind her, so she quickly leaned out her car window and signed her name.

"Thank you so much," the lady said. "My husband won't believe this when I tell him."

Mine won't either, Cristy thought as she waved goodbye and rounded the corner. She had to laugh. Of all the places to sign an autograph. She was delighted that people were so receptive to the record, though. Even with her new release, "I Have A Dream," out on the Liberty label, the new name for United Artists, "One Day At A Time" was still selling. She had even received her first gold record award from New Zealand.

Perhaps she'd even get to tour that country one day, now that the kids were grown. Tammy worked at the office as Lee's secretary and every now and then Cindy helped out part-time. Kevin worked at Madison Hospital as a pharmaceutical assistant. They all lived at home and could take care of themselves.

That made it so much easier to enjoy her trips with Lee and her band, "The Company." Daniel was performing with the show again, and Anne Marie was singing backup vocal. Cristy smiled as she thought about the girl who had been with her now for three years. She had joined the group in 1979, and they had become best friends. The guys on the bus must really get a kick out of the way the two of them could chatter for hours as they rolled down the highway, she thought. They would cover everything from what new book they were each reading to what new restaurant might be worth trying for lunch one day.

Cristy pulled into her driveway. She was surprised to see a frown on Lee's face as he came out to help her unload the groceries. Usually he was always so cheery and the one to keep her spirits up.

"Something the matter, Lee?" she asked.

"I'm so angry," he said as he reached into the car for a bag and began carrying it into the house. " 'I Have A Dream' was doing great until today. *Billboard* dropped your bullet. I couldn't believe it, especially after all the great comments I've been getting on the song."

He thought of all the people he had talked to in the past couple of weeks about the record. Lee Ranson, music director of WXCL in Peoria, had said it was just what the people needed during these rough times. He had added that it was a good positive, uplifting song and one of their most requested. Tim Byrd of WHK in Cleveland stated he thought it was a number one record the first time he heard it. Terry Moses of WIL in St. Louis commented that Cristy was also one of their most requested artists and Don Foster of CKLW in Winsor, Detroit had called "I Have A Dream" a stirring song.

Tommy Edwards of Record Haven in Cleveland even said he thought Cristy had another song of the year. Lee shook his head. It didn't make sense.

"So what happened?" Cristy asked, trying to hide her disappointment.

"When I called *Billboard*, they said it was an error due to computer breakdown. Do you believe it!"

"That doesn't sound fair. Can't they correct it in next week's issue?"

"No, it's too late. Stations have already started backing off it. It just makes me so mad when a legitimate record dies because of something like this," Lee said.

Cristy sighed. It took a lot to get Lee upset but she really couldn't blame him today after all his hard work. The only other time he had reacted like this was when WPLO in Atlanta quit playing her records. Lee figured it was because she did not do a station appreciation concert for them. She did several benefits a year for various organizations, including the Variety Club Telethon in St. Louis, and Lee had planned for her to do the show in Atlanta. But when they said she could only do ten minutes, Lee told them she wouldn't be able to make it. It would have been worth it if they could have done a thirty minute show, as originally planned, even though it would have cost him $2,000 personally for expenses. But Lee couldn't see making the trip for only ten minutes on stage. It wouldn't have been fair to Cristy.

Even though WPLO had quit playing her records, it hadn't hurt sales a bit. Her "One Day At A Time" album had sold over 50,000 copies in the Atlanta market area so far and was still going strong.

"Well, there's nothing we can do about it," Cristy said as she began to put the groceries away. She hated to see Lee like this. It bothered him much more than it did her. She looked over at her husband as he went over to his briefcase and pulled out some papers. Something else was on his mind, she could tell. Usually he didn't brood over things he couldn't change.

"Honey, is something else the matter?" she asked cautiously.

Lee kept his eyes on his paperwork. "I talked to Costello today. He told me he appealed the case to the US Circuit Court of Appeals in Chicago. Nine federal judges were scheduled to study his written argument against the RICO Act's application. Two judges excused themselves from the case altogether and the others, after studying the brief, ordered Mike and the attorneys for Martin and the sheriff to appear in court for oral arguments." Lee paused for a minute and leaned back in his chair at the kitchen table. "One judge wanted to know why I was even included in the government's case."

"And what happened?" Cristy asked quietly. Suddenly she was frightened. Lee had been so sure since his sentencing that he would not have to serve any time that she had believed him herself. Now she was not so sure.

"The panel upheld the conviction. Then Mike had to appeal it to the Supreme Court." Lee hesitated. "The Supreme Court turned down the appeal."

"Oh, no! Isn't there anything Mike can do?" she asked.

"Mike asked the judge to allow him to file a Rule 35 motion. It's based mostly on compassion. He will ask the judge to consider a suspension of active serving time or at least a reduction of the three years given," Lee explained. "He said he still thinks the judge will give me probation."

"And if he doesn't?" Her voice was strained as she spoke.

Lee stood up and walked over to his wife. He put his arms around her. "Now Cristy, that's not going to happen. At the worst, I might have to spend a day or two at the Maxwell Air Force Base in Alabama. They have a Federal Prison Camp there that Mike says is like a country club. No walls. No guns. Golf. Swimming pool and tennis. I would take a few days and just relax until Mike gets the whole thing cleared up." Lee made light of the situation but on the phone he had told Mike he did not want to go to any kind of prison. He knew there was no one who could handle things for Cristy's career. And worst of all would be having to be away from Cristy and the kids.

He had even prepared Tammy at the office just in case. "Tammy, we need to talk about what might happen," he had said.

"I don't want to consider that, Dad."

"We have to talk about it. I don't think I'm going to go anywhere, but we have to be prepared. I'm 44 years old now, and I've worked hard all my life. I've always tried to lead a good, honest life."

"I know you have," she said, fighting back the tears in her eyes.

Lee had to look away as he spoke, his own voice tight with emotion. "Since I was a young teen-ager and went to work on my own, I have been able to control where I would go and what I would do. This is a strange feeling for me—to know that another man, the judge, can say whether I'll be free or in prison, whether I can be here with my family or will have to go away. I don't like it, but we have to accept the situation."

"You won't have to go to prison, I know it!" she had said. "They don't put innocent people in prison. And you're innocent!"

"But, honey, if I do have to go, you stay close to your mother. We've already booked show dates six months in advance. Harold will be here to run the business and help you. You can handle the office end of things. And I know that you can comfort your mother at home. You're a strong girl, Tammy, and I'm proud of you."

Later, as he held Cristy in his arms, he tried to push away the sense of foreboding that had begun to gnaw at him. He did not tell any of his fears to Cristy. He didn't have to. He could already feel her trembling slightly in his arms.

* * *

When the day came for Lee to appear in court for the hearing in Springfield, Cristy insisted on going with him. The children, especially Tammy, wanted to go, but Lee refused.

Cristy was determined to be strong as she sat behind Lee and his attorney in the courtroom. There were only a few spectators, but the news media was represented by the TV networks and news agencies. She tried to push them out of her mind as she silently said a prayer for her husband.

He's been with me for almost twenty-three years, God, she prayed. Please don't let them take him away from me now. Then she watched the judge's face closely, hoping for some sign of encouragement as Lee took the stand.

"I did not give the sheriff ten percent of the money as that man Stone testified," Lee stated emphatically. "I am an innocent man."

The judge looked at Lee appraisingly before he explained that the hearing was not called to discuss the jury's verdict, but to consider a sentence reduction. He asked Lee how much of Cristy's career he handled.

"I work all areas—from promotion to production to booking, management, and even driving the bus."

"Will her career be able to continue on if you go to prison?"

Lee thought about his answer and replied honestly. He knew Cristy's name was secure in the music field. "It would suffer some, but we would find ways to carry on."

The judge looked toward Cristy and for a minute, she felt a surge of hope.

Costello addressed the court, saying that even "if everything said against Mr. Stoller were true, even if the testimony of Stone was accurate, he is the victim and not the guilty party in extortion. He would be as much a victim as any of those dozen or so others who came in and testified at the trial."

When the U.S. Attorney had his opportunity to speak, he criticized Lee for not taking the immunity offer. "Stoller had his chance. He wouldn't cooperate when he could. I think Stoller got a fair sentence of three years imprisonment. He bribed a public official, and he refused to be a witness for us."

Cristy could almost hear the door slam as the judge nodded his head. "Yes," he said, "that is a serious offense, bribing a public official."

The judge ordered a recess while he considered the testimony. Cristy fought to hold her composure when he returned and began to speak.

"Mr. Stoller, at this time I am going to rule out straight probation. The jury found you guilty, and it is my duty to serve the public in my capacity with the verdict handed down. I do feel a three-year sentence may be too severe, and I will keep your Rule 35 plea under advisement. But there will be no probation at this time."

Cristy cried silently as the judge ordered Lee to report to the Federal prison camp at Maxwell Air Force Base in Alabama within three weeks.

25

She and Lee had planned a quiet, intimate evening at one of their favorite oriental restaurants. But even the wonton soup she usually loved tasted bland tonight.

"Lee I want to cancel the show on May 14," she said hesitantly. "I want to be with you when you go in." It was still not easy for her to say the word "prison."

"Don't be silly. I want you to go on with your schedule as planned. Besides, Mike is still pushing that rule thirty-five. By the time I get there, the papers will probably be waiting to turn me loose." He chuckled reassuringly. "It'll be like a revolving door. I'll check in and check out. Cindy and Tammy can drive me down and probably bring me back."

She tried to smile as she looked across the table at her husband in the dimly lit room. She had found herself staring at him repeatedly these last few weeks as though he were going to disappear if she took her eyes off him. There was just too much to remember: the way the lines crinkled around his eyes when he laughed, the way he teased her, and even his endless chatter about the music business, no matter where they were. She would miss every irritating and wonderful thing about him.

She thought she was all cried out by now, but she supposed not as her eyes began to sting. It wasn't like she wouldn't be able to see him, she told herself, she would be able to visit him for several hours on weekends and holidays. But, she would be touring most weekends from now until November; and a visit just wasn't the same as having him home.

She had tried so hard not to be depressed around Lee and the kids. Lee kept saying, "Mike says it's like a country club. If it takes a day or two to get my release papers in order, I'll just relax and take life easy. Don't worry about me."

But she did worry. She knew Lee had always been his own person, working hard and making his own way in the world. No matter how nice the "club" was, she knew the hardest thing for him would be not to work; and to have someone else tell him how he had to fill his days.

Perhaps it would be best after all, if she didn't see him off. She had a feeling it would be worse for him if she were there. Cristy pushed back her plate of food, avoiding Lee's eyes as she spoke. "Can we go home now?"

"Sure, baby," Lee said. He looked at his own half-filled plate. "I'm not very hungry either."

Tammy, Cindy, and Lee got an early start the day he was to report to the prison camp. It was a five-and-a-half-hour drive south to Montgomery, Alabama, and Lee kept the atmosphere light and airy as they drove. He sat with his briefcase open on his lap half the way, going through last-minute details with Tammy about the office and what she and Harold needed to concentrate on.

When they reached Maxwell Air Force Base, the air policeman at the gate asked them their destination.

"The prison camp," Lee replied.

Tammy winced.

They drove past the military installation, past a small arms firing range and a golf course that encircled the camp. Tammy and Cindy followed as he walked into the bright, clean-looking administration building, briefcase in hand. It looked more like a military facility than a prison, Lee thought as he approached the reception area.

"I'm here to report in," he said to the small, conservatively-dressed woman behind the counter.

"What's your name?"

"Leland Stoller."

She surveyed him closely. Her eyes landed on his briefcase. "What's that you have with you?" she asked sharply.

"My business and personal things."

"You can't take that in with you," she remarked briskly.

"But it has all my paperwork and . . ."

"You may keep your shaving kit. You won't be needing anything else," she interrupted.

Lee felt like he was giving up a little piece of himself as he handed his briefcase to Cindy. She stood there, and suddenly it dawned on her that they actually were going to take him. She began to cry. She had really believed that he was going to simply check in and that he would be coming home with them.

Lee hugged both his daughters. "Take care of your mom. And don't worry," he said. "I won't be here long." He took a last look at their forlorn faces and turned to follow one of the correctional officers toward another stucco building.

He was led to a small "receiving and discharge" room at the camp's control center. His civilian clothes were taken away, and his naked body was checked for any contraband before he received his initial prison attire—a dull yellow jumpsuit with a zipper up the front. He was told he was allowed one civilian change of clothing. Another inmate led Lee to E Dormitory where he would be staying. He had been there less than an hour, and already he felt stripped of his dignity.

The first thing he did was find the telephone booths. He was allowed to make collect calls only and he was anxious to reach Mike Costello.

"What's happening with the judge, Mike? This could seriously damage Cristy's career if I have to stay in this place. It's going to cost me a fortune every day I'm away from business."

"Be calm, Lee. I'm sure the judge is going to reduce your sentence. Monday, first thing, I'll see him and try to get the word. You may be out of there in a matter of days."

Lee hung up the phone and sighed. He knew he wouldn't be able to reach Cristy until tomorrow since she was on the road. He decided he might as well get settled into his new quarters.

The dormitory was a clean, well-ventilated stucco building with bunks for over forty people. The bunks were divided into cubicles, white laminated wood circling each and standing almost eye level with an opening to the aisle. One row stood against each wall and two rows were back to back in the center.

Seniority determined who got the top bunk, the bottom bunk, or a private "cube." Since Lee was brand-new, he took the top bunk assigned to him and began to make up his bed, military style, with the blanket he'd been given. Then he carried his personal effects to the faded gray wall locker in a room at the front of the dorm near the bathrooms. He counted four showers and a line of sinks on one side and four commodes and a row of urinals on the other.

He walked around the grounds where he saw men picking up trash and sweeping the walk. This was a work camp, he had been told, and he would be assigned a job as soon as he finished orientation in a week. He found the recreation building, a clean masonry structure with three pool tables, a Ping Pong table, a music room, and a weight room with a scale. There was even a softball field with a game in progress between two dorms.

It wasn't until he climbed up in his bunk that night and tried to shut his eyes against the loud snoring and restlessness of forty other men that the full impact of his imprisonment hit him. This was no country club, and he wanted out.

The next morning orientation began. It was there he learned about the prison camp and followed the other new inmates as they were given a tour of the grounds.

The prison camp was first established in 1930. It was moved twice before settling in its present location bounded by the Alabama River on one side and the Air Force Base golf course on the other three. Just to the left of the camp entrance was a visitor's parking lot, adjacent to a large building used for administration and for an auditorium. Inmates gathered there for movies and other functions and to meet with their loved ones on weekends and holidays. Connected to the auditorium on one end was an outside visiting area enclosed by a chain link fence.

The second building held "control" where the officer on duty operated the radio and public address system. He was locked inside a room which faced the compound through heavy glass windows. Just inside the front door was the captain's office with two holding cells, used for disciplinary or transfer cases, beside it. Another room was used for "r & d" where mug shots were made, fingerprints taken and personal belongings surveyed. Unauthorized items were shipped home, and authorized packages sent in came through this facility.

Offices in the building included the physician's assistant and the dentist, along with quarters for case management where an inmate's file, progress and future release date were charted. There was also a small barbershop for inmates and an office for the chaplain. At the end of the building, facing the chain link fence, was a laundry room for the prison population: four rental washers and dryers which, Lee found out later, seldom worked.

There were seven dormitories, listed A through G. Six of them sat facing each other across a median of shrubbery and grass with sidewalks stretching parallel from the control building to the chow hall at the rear. The seventh dormitory sat doglegged to the left. On the other side of the kitchen was the education building with its law library, as required by federal edict, and classrooms.

In the rear of the compound were buildings for a welding class, mechanical services which kept the facilities in repair, and a warehouse where clothing and other supplies were stored and dispensed. Another building housed compound maintenance tools like shovels, brooms and rakes.

During orientation, Lee also learned the warden's feelings about the camp and its inmates.

"I have a closed door policy. I do not want any of you coming to see me about anything," R.D. Brewer said. "If you have a problem, go to my staff." Occasionally, the balding man could be seen sauntering daintily around the grounds as though he was inspecting his country estate. If he saw the inmates at all, it was by accident.

When Lee reached Cristy that afternoon, he knew all he ever wanted to know about the prison camp.

"Get a hold of Mike and get me outta here," he said, exasperated.

Cristy stifled a sob as she tried to sound cheerful. For him to say something like that, she knew he had to be miserable. "Have you heard anything at all?"

"When I talked to him yesterday he said he

would see the judge on Monday and that it shouldn't take more than a week to wrap things up. I sure hope he's right! How did the show go last night?"

"Okay," Cristy answered. "But it's not the same without you, Lee. I am so used to the way you handle everything. If we didn't need the money, I'd just as soon cancel the whole tour."

"Now, Cristy. It's really better that you stay busy. Besides, too many people are counting on you. I guess Tammy and Cindy got back all right. And how's Kevin?" Lee smiled as he thought of his eighteen-year-old son who had just gotten married. He was proud of him, out on his own. He'd seemed happy the last time they'd talked.

"He's just fine. I think he's worried about me, though. He's been over twice since you left."

"I'm glad he stops by. With just you and the girls there, I worry."

"Are they treating you all right? Do you get enough to eat?"

Lee chuckled at her worries. "Yes. The food's okay. That's one of the few nice things I can say about this place. I think it's run by idiots who think everyone else is an idiot like them."

"You're not in any danger, are you? I mean, from the other inmates."

"No, honey. Most of the people here are for non-violent, white collar crime. And it surprises me that there are a lot of other innocent people sent to prison for crimes they never committed. The system is all screwed up."

"Lee, I'm not concerned with the system right now, I just want to be sure you are okay. I'll be down to see you next Saturday. After the Friday night show, I'll fly to Nashville and drive down Saturday morning. I should be there by noon."

"When you see this place, maybe you won't be so worried," Lee said. "It's not as bad as you've pictured it, I'm sure."

Cristy drove up to the white stucco building for visitors at the Maxwell Camp. She had been averaging about three performances a week and on her days off she was usually very tired. But today she was too excited about seeing Lee to notice. She parked the car in the gravel lot and pulled out the cooler she had packed with all of Lee's favorite snacks. She had even baked him some of her oatmeal cookies. She knew he couldn't keep them but at least he could enjoy them for the few hours they would have together today and tomorrow. She had already made plans to spend the night at the Holiday Inn nearby.

As she walked into the reception area, she was surprised that there weren't any walls or guards with guns. She approached the desk, and the female guard immediately recognized Cristy from her TV album and complimented her on her music. Her name was Ms. Webster, and she was all smiles as she

examined the contents of the cooler while Cristy
filled out the visitors' form.

"I must check your pocketbook, too," she said as
Cristy started to walk away.

"Oh. Okay," Cristy said as she handed over her
purse and watched as the guard pulled out its contents item by item.

"What's this?" She held up a bottle of pills.

"My vitamins," Cristy replied.

"How do I know that? They could be anything."

"They are just my vitamins, really."

"I'm sorry," she said curtly. "If you want to go
in for a visit, you have to take them back out to your
car."

Cristy felt the blood rising in her cheeks as she
took the bottle and walked out to the car. She could
have been a little bit nicer about it, she thought.
How was she to know what was allowed and what
was not?

When she returned, Lee was paged. She had to
struggle to keep from running to him when he
came through the door. He looked a little thinner
to her and she held him tightly for as long as she
dared in plain view of all the other inmates and
their visitors. The auditorium was not exactly private but they managed to find a table in the back
where they could hold hands and kiss every now
and then.

"I feel just like a high school girl on a date with

a chaperon," Cristy said, eyeing the guard who sat at the elevated desk surveying the auditorium.

"They don't want anyone getting carried away," Lee said. "I'm just glad to have you next to me."

"I know. This week away from you has been like an eternity."

"Tell me about the show. How is it going?"

"As well as could be expected without you. The audiences have been really nice. It just seems so empty for me to sing without you there."

"It won't be long, sweetheart. Are you having any problems setting up and moving from show to show?"

"Anne Marie has been a great help there. She has been a real brick wall for me to lean on. Anne takes charge when we get to a show site, gets the band moving and ready to go. When it's over the band loads up the equipment while she wraps up the contracts with the show's sponsor. Annie is always there. When I'm depressed, she tries to cheer me up. When I have a problem and want to talk, which is often, she's there to listen."

"We're lucky honey, having both a true friend like Annie there, and Ken to do the driving."

"Lee, I don't understand why the judge doesn't do something about your sentence. If the courts realize you don't belong here, why can't they turn you loose?"

"The jury found me guilty," Lee shrugged. "They heard all the accusations against the sheriff and Martin and in their minds they associated me with it, even though I didn't know it was going on."

"But there was no evidence against you and the only witness against you was a known perjurer. I cannot believe a jury with any intelligence could find you guilty. Besides, judges have power. Why doesn't he do something?"

"I guess judges, even federal judges, have to consider public opinion, too. There was so much media coverage of the trial that he must feel he would be criticized if he did anything for me now. Your name was spread across the front pages around Missouri and Illinois."

"Even if he does nothing, you won't have to serve three years, will you?"

"Oh, no. I go to the parole board in July. The judge did give me a B-2 sentence which means the board can release me any time. Now if I had an 'A' sentence, which is a regular adult sentence, the board couldn't cut my time to less than one third of what the judge gave. Even if the judge doesn't release me before July I'm sure the board soon will."

"I certainly hope so."

Cristy stood up and began to unfold the red and white tablecloth she had brought. "I thought you might like a few things from home," she said as she carefully laid out the food and the china teacups she had packed.

As they ate, Lee introduced Cristy to several people who came up to her and wanted autographs.

People from all walks of life were there, he told her. Some of their families were wealthy but many had been left practically destitute due to lawyers and court costs and fines.

Cristy watched painfully as one little boy clung to his father's neck while the mother tried to pry him away. He couldn't understand why daddy couldn't go home with them.

"It's not as hard on us in here," Lee said, "as it is on you and the families. We're taken care of. There are some minor harassments, but that's nothing. When the courts put us away, they took the problems off our shoulders and put them on the families left at home."

"I guess that's something to be thankful for. At least we have enough saved up to get us through while you're in here," Cristy said.

"I know. The courts can be cold and impersonal. A man told me the other day how he knew he was coming to prison and he had several companies which he wanted to put in order before coming in, for his family. All he wanted was three weeks to sell what he had and leave his wife with some stability. The judge ordered him to be locked up the day he was sentenced. The mortgage company took their home which was only one payment overdue. People took over his companies and left his family with nothing. His wife had a nervous breakdown and had to go to a mental health center."

Cristy shook her head. "That's awful. There really ought to be a better way."

"One guy I talked to had a pretty good idea. He thinks that instead of putting white collar criminals in a jail where they can learn how to become better criminals, the judges ought to use community service as punishment. The lawbreaker could stay at home and do something constructive. Only if a man is a violent criminal should he be locked up.

"As it is now, crime nationwide is about a $200 billion dollar a year business, including everything from petty thefts to court costs," Lee said.

"Well, it's obvious this system isn't working. Is there really such a thing as rehabilitation?" Cristy asked.

"The Bureau of Prisons years ago admitted there is no rehabilitation in prison. That's just something they feed the public. If a man comes in here believing in the law, this experience would just turn him around. In fact, a large percentage of people are here because of entrapment. The government sets up crime situations, lures people into it with promises of quick money, and then arrests them."

"That doesn't sound legal to me," Cristy said skeptically.

"The courts every year take away more and more of people's rights," Lee insisted. "They catch a lot of guilty people but they admit that two out of three get away. And, unfortunately, a lot of innocent people are caught up in the system. Prosecutors look to make headlines and judges are seldom impartial, as they should be. It's more as if they are partners in the prosecution. And too many lawyers don't know the law like they should and aren't really qualified to represent their clients."

"Don't they have some sort of program to help inmates get back on their feet?"

"If a guy can't read or write, they teach him that here. That's about the extent of prisons contribution, though. The only program I've seen in prison that has benefits is recreation. It does teach the guys how to compete in sports together and that should help some of them get along with others. Besides that, it's a great escape valve. Just being here is so frustrating and the sports help blow off some steam."

Cristy stood up and began to put the food away. She noticed with dismay that Lee hadn't eaten very much. "How are the guards?" she asked, wanting to lighten the conversation.

"Some are pretty good. There are people here like Susan James, Yancy, Davis, Hudson, and Harry Long who do their job but still treat us as if we're human beings. Some of the others act as if we crawled out from under a rock."

Cristy thought of the guard she'd met on her way in that afternoon and she knew exactly what Lee meant.

"A staff member told me that the prison bureau

was the bottom of the barrel and got stuck with the worst personnel in the Justice Department." Lee laughed sarcastically. "Some of these guys couldn't get a job in a pie factory."

Cristy looked at her husband searchingly. Sometimes his bravado could get him in trouble. She just wanted this whole ordeal to be over and for him to come home. "You will be careful, won't you, Lee? You won't let any of this change you?" she asked apprehensively.

"Of course not. I'll be fine."

It wasn't easy for Cristy to smile the next day when she kissed Lee goodbye. She promised him that Cindy or Tammy or Kevin would be down to visit him on the weekend that she would be on the road.

As the auditorium began to clear out, Lee clung to her as if he couldn't bear the thought of her leaving. The hardest part for Cristy was when she thought she saw tears in his eyes as he turned to follow the other inmates back to their dorm. She had never seen her husband cry before.

Days became weeks and weeks slowly turned into months as Lee continued to serve time. He called Cristy every day and kept in contact with Tammy and Harold to advise them on business matters as best he could. He was constantly on the phone to Costello and his attorney always said the same thing, "We should get word any day now."

He fought bitterness about being at the camp at

all and he forced himself to be optimistic. He would tell himself and anyone who'd listen, "I'll be out of here by the end of the week." He joined the softball team and when he came up to bat he was often serenaded with a take off of Cristy's song "Lee's serving time, One Day At A Time."

He was assigned a job as groundskeeper for the warden. He gradually met the other residents at the camp. There were lawyers and drug dealers, doctors and CPAs. Counterfeiters and tax offenders. Regardless of the charge, guilty or innocent, everyone was accepted for what he was at present and not for what he had been or what he had owned.

At first he was outgoing and friendly. But when an inmate started an argument, and threatened to kill him, Lee decided that he had better be more cautious about the company he kept.

He was surprised to learn that unlawful acts that would have been contemptible on the outside were praised in the camp. Some inmates boasted of theft and deception or talked about the other prisons where they had served time.

It was no wonder there were so many repeat offenders, Lee thought. Any kind of crime imaginable could be concocted from the knowledge among the inmates. It seemed to him, that the camp was more a school for crime than a correctional facility.

Lee never lost hope for an early release. But he sorely missed Cristy and traveling with her on the road. He talked about her to anyone and everyone who would listen, until finally he and the office managed to get her booked on the base for a benefit concert. The date was set for July 10th, three days after Lee was supposed to see the parole board. He was so excited until one thing after another almost convinced him to cancel the show entirely.

Cristy's brother, Raymond, was suddenly killed in an accident. He was driving his pickup truck just as her brother Charlie had been when he'd been killed. Lee was refused permission to go to the funeral. Camp policy, they said, included only immediate members of the family. A staff member confided to Lee that the administrators felt intimidated by wealthy or famous people and tried to make things harder for them.

Then, adding insult to injury, the parole board gave him a sentence of fourteen months instead of a much lighter sentence they would have given, if the correct information had been put on his PSI (personal sheet of information). The bureau used rigid guidelines in determining the length of time to be served. Lee's time was set for fourteen to twenty-four months, when it should have read ten to fourteen.

Finally, when Lee tried to get permission for the inmates to see Cristy's show, he was turned down. The warden said Cristy was a professional and that her husband was serving time; consequently no one was allowed to go. Many of the inmates considered his decision a cruel and heartless one for other inmates' wives were allowed to sing on camp at church.

Several days before the show, Tammy asked Lee if he wanted them to cancel the show. He said, "Go ahead with it. These Air Force guys deserve it, even if this warden wants to punish the inmates and deprive them of some entertainment."

There was an empty feeling inside Cristy as she stepped on stage the night of the performance at Maxwell Air Force Base. The news of her brother's death had devastated her, and the thought that Lee was so close, and yet unable to be with her made her feel lonelier than ever.

She performed her entire show confidently, somehow masking the ache she felt inside. When she came to her last song, however, she changed the introduction. Usually she began "One Day At A Time" by saying, "With all the turmoil in the world today, perhaps the answer lies in this song." But tonight, she simply said, "This is for my husband, Lee Stoller."

When she got to the chorus of the song, she knew she could not keep up the facade any longer. She stopped singing as a lump rose in her throat and tears began to sting her eyes. She bent her head and swallowed hard. She was so embarrassed but it was no use, she couldn't finish the song.

The band continued to play as she walked off the

stage. Cindy had been watching from the audience and she met her mother as she stepped off the platform. She put her arms around her and held her as she spoke, "We'll have him home soon, Mom. We'll have him home soon."

26

*C*risty wondered how she had made it through the last year. It had been the longest and loneliest time of her life. And things at the office had not gone very well. They lost both records that were released in the past year on Cristy from the lack of proper promotion. Cristy felt her career had been stalemated.

As she drove the now familiar road to Montgomery, Alabama, this Thursday afternoon, the thought ran through her mind: They say God never gives you more trouble than you can handle. Well, she smiled inwardly, it seems He's certainly had a field day with me in my lifetime!

But He had never been more than a prayer away, she realized, from the time she was a little girl till now. He was there even when she was sure he couldn't possibly be listening.

Hadn't she acquired a sense of her own self-worth? She no longer trembled before anyone as she had once before a preacher who told her she was unworthy. And she no longer felt the cruel sting of other people's laughter as she had the night her teacher turned her away because of her dress. Now if someone seemed to be laughing at her, she held her head up high, knowing that the other person had the problem, not she.

And hadn't she overcome her awful terror of singing before an audience? Her knees no longer knocked now, when she stood on stage, and more often than not, she even felt good about herself when she finished a show.

Surely, God had been with her in Vietnam. She had come close to death too often not to realize He had been with her every horrible day during those three months. And of course, He had given her Lee to love. Even though she'd thought at times that He had abandoned her during Lee's imprisonment, she realized now He had not. Instead, she had discovered a strength of character, a kind of mettle she had never known she'd possessed until she had been put to the test, as she had been this past year.

She had been forced to do things she'd never done before. She had had to handle business and money matters with Tammy and make contract and show decisions with Annie when they were on the road. She had gone to music functions and business dinners facing questions about Lee as Tammy stood by her side, trying to fill her father's shoes.

She sighed as she thought of her eldest daughter. Of all the children, Lee's absence had seemed to affect her the most. She had Lee's bravado and Cristy had been proud of her when she spoke up to the judge in Springfield when they had gone together to intercede for Lee on the Rule thirty-five. Later, she was surprised to learn that Tammy had even written a letter to the judge on her own, saying she thought it was unfair that her father, an innocent man, should be serving time. But the pressures at the office and the responsibilities she felt without her father around, had almost proved too much for her twenty-one years. She had become agitated and depressed, crying almost every day. Cristy thought her daughter was going to have a nervous breakdown, but possessing her father's fortitude, she'd fought it off.

Cristy had to be mother, father and confidante as she drove Tammy home one night just after they had gone out to eat. Her daughter had begun crying uncontrollably in the restaurant and Cristy's heart went out to her. She felt so helpless as she looked over at her daughter in the car. Finally she told her she would just have to try and get a hold of herself. "Why not start reading some self-help books and the Bible," she had said. "They helped me when I was not much older than you and they still do."

Time, talking and a lot of prayers had helped her see her daughter through those rough spots. She smiled when she recalled how much happier Tammy had seemed once the whole family was together at Thanksgiving.

Lee had received a five-day furlough, and the family spent it in Birmingham where Cristy was to do a benefit show to raise money for the Alabama Symphony Orchestra. Tammy, Cindy, Kevin and his wife Mary, Lee and Cristy were all together for the first time in months. They even got to celebrate Lee's birthday on November 26.

That had been a wonderful week, Cristy thought. A whole five days with Lee had been so much nicer than the occasional day passes Lee received when she would pick him up and spend a day together away from the camp. She shuddered when she thought about the indignities he had to suffer every time she brought him back to the camp in the evening. He had to strip naked while he was checked for contraband, take a urine test, and blow into a balloon-like device that determined whether or not he'd had any alcohol. Watching his crestfallen face as she pulled away from the camp was always the most painful part for her.

As the road whizzed by her she thought of the many miles she had covered during the summer and through November completing her tour dates without Lee by her side. They had always worked together and she had so loved the road trips with him. His constant bantering with the band members and his friendly, incessant chatter would fill the bus as he would pull into a "Mr. Donut" or search for a nice restaurant in a new town where everybody could enjoy a relaxed dinner. And no one emcee'd the shows as Lee could.

But Ken and the other drivers had driven the bus this past summer and she had spent most of her time in her room at the rear of the bus, reading and trying not to stare out the window. She had tried to put up a strong show of cheerfulness for the band. She didn't want anyone to pity her. She had been particularly glad for Annie, though. They didn't have to talk about it much, but Cristy could tell she sensed her loneliness and isolation. Just having her nearby was a great comfort. And she knew her friend had tried to ease the burden of traveling without Lee by handling as many details for the show and the band as possible.

Cristy breathed a sigh of relief as she turned into the Air Force Base and passed the sign, "Maxwell Prison Camp." Today was the last time she would ever have to see that sign.

It was February 3, 1983, as Lee Stoller sat on the banks of the Alabama River outside his dormitory.

He looked at his watch. Cristy should be here soon, he thought. He had been packed for hours—days, practically, since he'd learned of his release date.

For a while there, he had thought Mike would never get to see the judge to discuss the Rule thirty-five. First, the judge had hepatitis, then it was discovered he had cancer of the stomach and Mike had to wait until he was well enough to meet with him. The judge had reduced his sentence to a year and a day but that had seemed like forever to Lee, who had been confident he would be released "any day now." In December, he tried to get permission to be sent to a halfway house where he could at least be in Nashville and work at the office and be near his family.

When that was turned down, he tried not to be bitter or lose his perspective. At least he was getting out today. He frowned as he thought about one of the inmates who would never leave; his name was simply "Doc." He was a cheery person, who, it was said, had been in a car wreck that left him lame and had put a permanent indentation in his forehead.

Camp rumor said Doc was taking small boxes of cereal from prison mess and mailing them home to his family, and that he often hoarded pills from the clinic and dispensed them himself to other inmates. On one occasion, Doc had persuaded an ex-commissioner from Tennessee to take eight laxative pills to clear his system. The recipient of this free medical advice had spent several days going between the bathroom and the shower.

Everyone liked Doc and overlooked his pecularities. It was a surprise, though, when he'd been caught wrapping up a typewriter from the camp warehouse and trying to mail it home. The administration charged him with theft of government property and locked him in the hole, a small two-man cell in the control building.

During his confinement, when his cellmate was out in the visiting yard, Doc committed suicide. The story was he'd scraped his wrists on the rough edges of the bunk until he started bleeding and then stretched out on his bunk to die. The story went that Doc had been threatened with severe prosecution over the typewriter incident by the case manager, McSweeney, instead of being sent for proper psychiatric help.

One inmate even tried to interest the news media in the story but to no avail. People did not want to think about these places, Lee thought. He wished that just once judges, prosecutors, crooked lawyers and even jurors could spend a few days in prison to see what it was like. Perhaps then, they wouldn't be so quick to lock people up. He felt it would be better to let 100 guilty people go free than for the jury to convict one innocent person. And if you're ever on a jury consider the law, if a reasonable doubt exists you shouldn't vote guilty.

The whole system seemed fouled up to Lee. Here he was, an innocent man, serving a year and a day, on a three-year sentence, when Martin, who had been given fifteen years, would be free in just eleven months. Well, at least, Lee said to himself,

I've been given time off for good behavior. To date,
I've actually been in the camp for eight months and
twenty days instead of the full twelve months. Finally I'm going home.

Lee got up to stretch. He noticed his pants slipping again and he pulled his belt a notch tighter.
That was one good thing, he thought wryly; he'd
lost the paunch he had acquired over the years of
sitting behind a desk. His job at the camp, which
had been changed from groundskeeper to Gymna-
sium Clerk had kept him busy as did the softball
team and other sports.

He was looking forward to getting back behind
the desk again. He was frustrated by the lack of
promotion of Cristy's career during the past year.
He produced another television album to be
released on her. It was called "Heart Touching
Songs" and promotion was just starting to get
under way. And he was finishing the book he had
always wanted to have written about Cristy.

He smiled as he thought of his wife. He was so
proud of her. To think the girl he had been married
to for six years before he even knew she could sing,
now held five gold and three platinum record
awards from Canada, New Zealand, and the U.S.
And Lee had a surprise for her. He had a very
special plaque made up by a prisoner. It was for
having the number one gospel album in the world,
over a million sold, "One Day At A Time."

She had come so far and he knew hers was a

unique story of personal growth and triumph over her own fears and self-doubt. She had insisted, though, that the story be about both of them, since, she said, without his faith and management ability, she never would have sung at all. She had also insisted that the book be honest. "If so much about me is going to be revealed, I want it to be the truth," she had said. "Perhaps then it can be a source of hope and inspiration for others. You're the only one that can write it."

Lee walked into his dorm and gathered up his bags. He would not miss this place, he thought, and it wouldn't be easy facing some of the people who knew where he had been. Even though he was innocent, there were bound to be those who would wonder. He had even kept the news from his father who had been in poor health the past couple of years. Lee had simply told him he was in seclusion working on Cristy's book.

Of all the things he'd learned though, the most important had been realizing how much his family meant to him. All the gold records, the fame and the fortune could not buy what he had with Cristy and the children. He wanted to slow down a bit now; maybe get a place in Florida or California where he and Cristy could spend some time together.

He could never have gotten through this ordeal without her by his side. She had always been there for him: through his infidelity, his job changes, his sometimes insensitivity to her fears of performing,

the horrors of Vietnam, and now his imprisonment. That shy little eighteen-year-old girl he had
fallen in love with one night at the roller skating
rink had proved to be a pillar of strength.

Lee smiled and waved as he saw Cristy's car pull
up to the front of the administration building. He
was a lucky man.

Cristy waved back as she got out of the car. She
felt like a school girl on her first date again, and she
laughed at herself as her heart beat with happy
expectation. He still has that irrepressible smile,
she thought. And there is still that familiar bounce
in his step.

It seemed to her she had never loved him as much
as she did at this moment. She whispered a silent
prayer of thanks as Lee took her in his arms.

Lee whispered in her ear, "I thank God and you
for my life."

They headed back to Nashville, neither of them
exactly sure what the future held in store . . . yet
both oddly high . . . uptempo . . . it was a strange
feeling . . . like one of victory . . . as though this were
a brand-new day beginning for them, and nothing
could stop them, no matter what . . . they were
together, and they would take it together . . . one
day at a time . . .

A SPECIAL DEDICATION TO THE BRAVE U.S. SERVICEMEN WHO SO OFTEN ARE FORGOTTEN.

It is with love, respect and gratitude that I dedicate the following prayer to all veterans who so unselfishly served our country in times of war.

The Lord's Prayer has meant so very much to me throughout my life. It has given me strength to carry on; the same strength it must have taken for our fighting men to press forward to victory. It gives comfort in times of distress, relief in affliction, and reassurance when disheartened. All of these problems, I am certain, have been shared by anyone who has faced the tragedies of war.

I can never forget the thousands of young smiling faces I saw while touring Viet Nam to entertain our servicemen. I will always remember the courage and strength they displayed although fighting in a thankless conflict. They have a special place in my heart.

Above all, I dedicate this prayer in loving remembrance of those who made the supreme sacrifice of their lives so that we might continue to live a free people.

God Bless You All,

Cristy

THE LORD'S PRAYER

Our father which art in heaven
Hallowed be thy name

Thy kingdom come thy will be done
On earth as it is in heaven

Give us this day our daily bread
And forgive us our debts
As we forgive our debtors

And lead us not into temptation
But deliver us from evil

For thine is the kingdom and the power
And the glory, forever
Amen.

AWAY IN A MANGER

Away in a manger, no crib for a bed
The little Lord Jesus, laid down his sweet
head
The stars in the sky, looked down where he
lay
The little Lord Jesus asleep on the hay

The cattle are lowing the baby awakes
But little Lord Jesus no crying he makes
I love thee, Lord Jesus, look down from the
sky
And stay by my cradle till morning is nigh

Be near me Lord Jesus, I ask thee to stay
Close by me forever, and love me I pray
Bless all the dear children in thy tender
care
And take us to heaven to live with thee
there

The first song Cristy sang at Church.

GOD'S WHISPER

"Anybody might have heard it, but God's whisper came to me," says the poet.

God always whispers. At least to the soul. He may thunder to nations and speak to armies in the lightning. But to the individual His message is not in the mighty wind, nor the earthquake, nor the fire, but in the still small voice.

God lives in the bottom of the funnel of silence. He is the treasure concealed in solitude. He meets men alone, in the dark. Congregations have their use, and books, and papers, and multitudes, and friends, but God loves the silent way.

He is every soul's most secret secret. If, as Thoreau said, it takes two to tell the truth, it also takes two to make a revelation; it takes the whisper of God and the listening of man.

God's whisper runs to and fro upon the earth. It might be heard in all cottages, palaces, marts, offices, inns and councils—if only we listened.

Go into the silence. Give your souls time to calm. Let the hurly-burly die down, the crash of passion, the struggle of doubt, the pain of failure, the ranklings of wrong, the clamor of ambition. Cease from self. Be still.

Practice this. It is an art, and not to be mastered out of hand. Try it again and again, as patiently, as determinedly, as lovingly as one practices the violin or the making of a statue.

And after awhile, as virtuosity comes after long trials, there will come to life in you the needed sixth sense, by which you can hear the whisper.

Some day you will get it. It may rise like a strange dawn in your consciousness. It may stir in you as life stirs in the egg. It may penetrate the deep chambers of your being as a strain of mystic music.

And it will be the prize of life. You will not be able to give it to another. Every man must receive such things himself. All of God's most vital secrets are marked nontransferable.

But it will be yours—that which in all your life is most utterly yours. It will strengthen you in weakness, cheer you in hours of gloom. When you are at sea and confused, lost in the winds of casuistry, it will shine out as a pole-star. When you are afraid it will reinforce you as an army with banners.

It will lull you to sleep with its music. It will give you poise. It will give you decision. No man can tell what the whisper says. Each soul must hear for itself. This is a great secret. One can only point the way—the way to silence.

There stands God and says: "I will give to eat of the hidden manna, and will give him a white stone, and in the stone a new name written, which no man knoweth saving he that receiveth it. He that hath an ear, let him hear what the Spirit saith."

(Anonymous)

THE BIBLE! THERE IT STANDS!

Where childhood needs a standard
    Or youth a beacon light,
Where sorrow sighs for comfort
    Or weakness longs for might,
Bring forth the Holy Bible,
    The Bible! There it stands!
Resolving all life's problems
    And meeting its demands.

Though sophistry conceal it,
    The Bible! There it stands!
Though Pharisees profane it,
    Its influence expands;

It fills the world with fragrance
Whose sweetness never cloys,
It lifts our eyes to heaven,
It heightens human joys.

Despised and torn in pieces,
By infidels decried—
The thunderbolts of hatred
The haughty cynics pride—
All these have railed against it
In this and other lands,
Yet dynasties have fallen,
And still the Bible stands!

LEE'S STUFFING

1 lb. bag Pepperidge Farm Stuffing
2 cups crushed crackers
1 cup onion
1 cup chopped green pepper
½ cup chopped celery
½ cup chopped carrots
1 jar (4½ oz.) mushrooms
1 cup chopped chicken giblets (cooked)
1 cup chopped chicken livers (cooked)
2 cloves minced garlic
3 pints oysters (uncooked)
1 tsp. sage
1 tsp. spiced salt
1 tsp. garlic salt
1 tsp. black pepper

1 tsp. hickory smoke salt
2 beaten eggs
¼ lb. butter melted in 1 cup hot water
(Watkins Spices are recommended)

Mix all ingredients in large bowl. Spoon into baking dishes. Bake uncovered for 1 hr. or till done to your liking. Bake at 325°.

CRISTY'S SHRIMP NEWBURG

1 lb. fresh or frozen shrimp in shells
4 tablespoons flour (all purpose)
4 tablespoons butter
2 cups milk
¼ cup Holland House Cooking Wine or your favorite white wine
2 tablespoons lemon juice
Patty shells or toast points

In large saucepan bring 1 quart of water and 3 tbsps. salt to boil. Add shrimp. Heat to boiling; reduce heat and simmer till shrimp turn pink, 1 to 3 minutes. Drain. Peel shrimp and remove black vein. Split peeled shrimp lengthwise.

In making the white sauce:

In medium saucepan melt 4 tablespoons butter; blend in the 4 tablespoons of flour till it's absorbed into the butter; let bubble for 1 minute. Remove from heat and stir in milk a little at a time till smooth. Return to medium heat and cook stirring constantly till thickened. You may want to add a little salt & pepper at this time plus the dry white wine. Stir in shrimp and lemon juice. (You may add other seafood to this dish.) Heat through. Serve on toast points or patty shells.

LEE'S FRIED RICE

1 box Fried Rice
4 beaten eggs
1 large potato
1 small onion, chopped
1 green pepper, chopped
1 clove garlic
1 jar 2½ oz. chopped mushrooms
1 can bean sprouts
1 tsp. spice salt
1 tsp. black pepper
3 tsp. soy sauce

Follow directions on box in preparing fried rice. Fry the potato, add onion, green pepper, mushrooms, bean sprouts, fried rice, eggs, spice salt, pepper, soy sauce.
Cook on low heat about 20 minutes.

CRISTY'S FESTIVE BAKED BEANS

1 can Big John's Beans & Fixin's
1 tsp. Grey Poupon Dijon Mustard
½ cup onion, diced

½ cup green pepper, diced
½ jar mushrooms, diced
1 small carrot, diced
1 tbsp. catsup
2 tablespoons brown sugar
1 tbsp. sherry cooking wine
1 clove minced garlic

In baking dish mix beans & fixin's and all ingredients listed. Top with slices of bacon or ham (fat trimmed off). Bake 350° oven 45 minutes or till done.

FOOTPRINTS IN THE SAND
By Daniel Willis

One night I had a dream—I dreamed I was walking along the beach with the Lord. And across the sky flashed scenes from my life. For each scene, I noticed two sets of footprints in the sand. One set belonged to me, and the other to the Lord.

When the last scene of my life flashed before us, I looked back at the footprints in the sand; I noticed that many times along the path of life, there was only one set of footprints: I also noticed that it happened at the very lowest and saddest times in my life. This really bothered me and I questioned the Lord about it.

One set of footprints in the sand
Lord you promised me you'd hold my hand
Tell me why in the troubled times
I look back and only find
One set of footprints in the sand

"Lord, you said that once I decided to follow you, you would walk with me all the way. But I have noticed that during the most troublesome times in my life, there is only one set of footprints. I don't understand why in times when I needed you most, you should leave me." The Lord replied, "My precious, precious child, I love you, and I would never,

never leave you during your times of trial and suffering. When you saw only one set of footprints in the sand, it was then I was carrying you."

One set of footprints in the sand
Oh, at last I understand
Through every storm he carried me
Now I praise the Lord each time I see
One set of footprints in the sand

*This is Cristy's version.

IN MEMORIAM

Pansy Johnston

October 18, 1903
May 26, 1986

To the greatest lady I've ever known, Pansy Johnston. She may never have seen her name in lights or won an Oscar or an Emmy. She just raised a family of twelve children through the great depression. Through the wars, all six of her boys served their country honorably.

Though she never had the luxuries nor money that most people did, God blessed her with the greatest gifts of all: a sense of humor, peace of mind, happiness, and love. She shared each of these gifts with everyone she knew.

And at the end of her long life's journey, at the age of eighty-two, she won the ultimate award. Thank you, Jesus, for opening up the gates of heaven for my dear mother. The memories she has blessed us with will be cherished forever.

Until we are reunited she shall always remain in my mind and heart.

Love forever from your daughter and family.

Eleanor Stoller
(Cristy Lane)

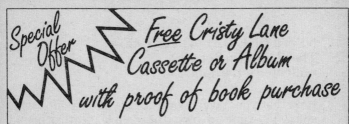

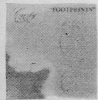

THE TALKING BOOK—
One Day at a Time
Narrated on Cassette Tapes

Cristy Lane's is such a great story that we now have *One Day at a Time—The Talking Book* available on a set of four cassette tapes. Enjoy Cristy Lane's life story, narrated by famous announcer Chris Lane. A perfect gift idea, The Talking Book comes with the following *free* bonus items:

- A copy of One Day at a Time, Cristy Lane's story told in pictures and text. A $10.99 value, it is yours *free* with the purchase of The Talking Book.

- The *One Day at a Time* soundtrack cassette tape. Including the number one hit, "One Day at a Time," and many others.

You can own the entire package: The Talking Book, a copy of *One Day at a Time*, and the cassette soundtrack, for only $19.95. Use the handy coupon below when ordering.

ORDER YOUR OWN
CRISTY LANE RECORD COLLECTION!

Cristy Lane—*Christmas Is the Man from Galilee*

Shake Me I Rattle • Pretty Paper • White Christmas • Jingle Bells • Silent Night • Joy to the World • Away in a Manger • The First Noel • Man from Galilee • What Child Is This • A Little Bit Colder • Upon the House Top • O Holy Night • It Came upon a Midnight Clear • O Little Town of Bethlehem • Jolly Old St. Nicholas • O Come, All Ye Faithful • Blue Christmas • Old Christmas Card • God Rest Ye Merry Gentlemen

Cristy Lane—*Harbor Lights*
A Masterpiece of the World's Greatest Love Songs

Harbor Lights • Fascination • Allegheny Moon • San Francisco • Believin' Your Love • Love Letters in the Sand • Smoke Gets in Your Eyes • Always on My Mind • More • It's Down to You and Me • Shadow of Your Smile • To Each His Own • Que Sera, Sera • Danny Boy

Cristy Lane—*Greatest Hits*
Twelve of Cristy's Most Popular Songs

One Day at a Time • Footprints in the Sand • I Have a Dream • Shake Me, I Rattle • Love Lies • Rainsong • Simple Little Words • Fragile, Handle with Care • Penny Arcade • Sweet Sexy Eyes • I Just Can't Stay Married to You • The Man from Galilee • Let Me Down Easy

---

Each Cristy Lane collection is available on albums, 8-track tapes, and cassettes.
Please rush me the following:
Christmas Is the Man from Galilee ($10.00 each) _____
Harbor Lights ($10.00 each) _____
Greatest Hits ($10.00 each) _____

Total _____

Please check one: ☐ Album(s) ☐ 8-Track(s) ☐ Cassette(s)
Send check or money order to LS Records, Cristy Lane, Dept. B, Madison, TN 37116, or:

Charge to my ☐ VISA ☐ MASTERCARD
☐ AMERICAN EXPRESS ☐ DINERS CLUB

Card No. _____ *Exp. Date* _____

Name _____

Address _____

City _____ *State* _____ *Zip* _____

$9.98 Cassette Free! When you buy the *Cristy Lane Doll*

Many have heard the voice and read the life story. Now you and your children can enjoy your very own replica of Cristy.

THE CRISTY LANE DOLL

This doll is an authentic replica of Cristy created by Horsman Dolls, Inc., from an actual life mask of Cristy's face. She is 14 inches tall, made from soft vinyl and polyethelene, and her head, arms, and legs are moveable. Her clothing is patterned after the actual garments worn by Cristy. Horsman Dolls, Inc., has been creating many of America's best known and loved dolls since 1865.

FREE CASSETTE OFFER—With the purchase of this doll you will receive absolutely *free* a cassette of Cristy Lane's *Simple Little Words*. Also included in this package is a birth certificate for your doll. A $9.98 value, yours for purchasing the Cristy Lane doll.

Simple Little Words features these ten songs:

- Simple Little Words
- Away in a Manger
- Upon the House Top
- Garden for a Special Friend
- He's Got the Whole World in His Hands
- Jesus Loves Me
- Turn Your Love Light On
- Everlasting Arms
- Under His Wing
- Lord's Prayer

BONUS OFFER! With your Cristy Lane doll's birth certificate, you are an *automatic winner!* Just present your ticket stub and birth certificate at a Cristy Lane concert and pick up a *free gift*—of your choice!

LS Records, Dept. Doll-1, 120 Hickory Street, Madison, TN 37115

Please rush me the beautiful Cristy Lane doll with birth certificate and my *free* cassette, *Simple Little Words*, on your unconditional money-back guarantee. I am enclosing $19.95 plus $3.00 shipping and handling.

Charge to my ☐ VISA ☐ MASTERCARD
☐ AMERICAN EXPRESS ☐ DINERS CLUB

Card No. _____ *Exp. Date* _____

Name _____
Address _____
City _____ *State* _____ *Zip* _____

Use your credit card, or send check or money order to:
LS Records, Dept. Doll-1, 120 Hickory Street, Madison, TN 37115

Christy Lane/One Day
At A Time T-Shirts

Standard

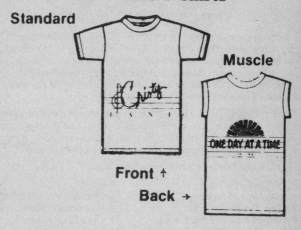

Muscle

ONE DAY AT A TIME

Front ↑

Back →

YES! Please rush me (_____) Cristy Lane T-Shirt(s). I have enclosed my check, or money order (U.S. Funds).

PLEASE CHECK (√) ITEMS WANTED BELOW:

_____Standard T-Shirt $10.00   ☐ Small
_____Muscle (sleeveless) T-Shirt $10.00 ☐ Medium
_____White   ☐ Large
_____Light Blue   ☐ X-Large
_____Raspberry
_____Aqua
_____Beige

PLEASE NOTE: The white T-shirt design consists of Cristy's photo on the front. All other colors consist of design shown.

**CES Marketing
P.O. Box 24504
Nashville, TN 37202**

Make checks payable to CES Marketing.
Tennessee residents please add 7.75% sales tax.
Please add $2.00 for shipping & handling.